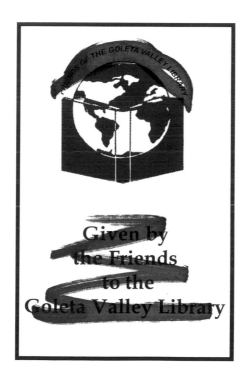

DIAGNOSING GIANTS

Diagnosing Giants

SOLVING THE MEDICAL MYSTERIES OF THIRTEEN
PATIENTS WHO CHANGED THE WORLD

Philip A. Mackowiak, MD, MBA, MACP

DIRECTOR, MEDICAL CARE CLINICAL CENTER
VA MARYLAND HEALTH CARE SYSTEM
PROFESSOR AND VICE CHAIRMAN, DEPARTMENT OF MEDICINE
UNIVERSITY OF MARYLAND SCHOOL OF MEDICINE
BALTIMORE, MD

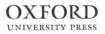
OXFORD
UNIVERSITY PRESS

OXFORD
UNIVERSITY PRESS

Oxford University Press is a department of the University of Oxford.
It furthers the University's objective of excellence in research, scholarship,
and education by publishing worldwide.

Oxford   New York
Auckland   Cape Town   Dar es Salaam   Hong Kong   Karachi
Kuala Lumpur   Madrid   Melbourne   Mexico City   Nairobi
New Delhi   Shanghai   Taipei   Toronto

With offices in
Argentina   Austria   Brazil   Chile   Czech Republic   France   Greece
Guatemala   Hungary   Italy   Japan   Poland   Portugal   Singapore
South Korea   Switzerland   Thailand   Turkey   Ukraine   Vietnam

Oxford is a registered trademark of Oxford University Press in the UK and certain other
countries.

Published in the United States of America by
Oxford University Press
198 Madison Avenue, New York, NY 10016

© Oxford University Press 2013

Library of Congress Cataloging-in-Publication Data
Mackowiak, Philip A.
Diagnosing giants : solving the medical mysteries of thirteen patients who
changed the world / Philip A. Mackowiak.
   p. ; cm.
Includes bibliographical references and index.
ISBN 978–0–19–993777–6 (alk. paper)
I. Title.
[DNLM: 1. Diagnosis. 2. Famous Persons. 3. Disease. 4. History of Medicine. WZ 313]
LC Classification not assigned
616.07′5—dc23
2012051224

9 8 7 6 5 4 3 2 1
Printed in the United States of America
on acid-free paper

To Connie
For love, happiness, and the support that made this book possible.

Contents

Preface

THIS BOOK, like its prequel, *Post Mortem: Solving History's Great Medical Mysteries*, traces the history of medicine through the illnesses of some of the most influential figures of the past. One might ask, why study history, or more precisely, why study the history of medicine? Surely there are more than enough facts related to the medicine of today to satisfy the thirst for medical knowledge of any physician or interested layperson. A lifetime of dedicated study could not even begin to master all of the many facets of the science of medicine as it exists at this very moment, much less the new concepts that like Pelion would be piled upon Ossa during the course of such study. Why, for that matter, would historians concern themselves with the history of medicine? Surely there are enough momentous political, sociological, religious, and military events to fully occupy their curiosity.

The answer, of course, is that what is past truly is prologue. Our yesterdays have determined who we are today, and knowledge of our past has the potential to enhance both our understanding of the present and enlighten our predictions of the future. Moreover, such knowledge is the ultimate antidote to the hubris that would have us believe that our generation's answers to life's great questions, medical and otherwise, are totally correct and truly our own.

But why, in particular, study the medical histories of people who in various ways influenced the course of human history? The answer is that in many cases their diseases had potentially profound effects on their lives as well as their legacies.

Moreover, standard biographies all too often pay scant attention to the health issues that affected their subjects. Such issues are interesting in their own right but also offer a unique opportunity to trace the evolution of medical concepts through their impact on the lives and accomplishments of extraordinary people just as they have influenced those of ordinary people like us.

Acknowledgments

I AM INDEBTED to a host of gifted clinicians, historians, librarians, artists, and scholars for the inspiration, the ideas, and the support that made possible this sequel to *Post Mortem: Solving History's Great Medical Mysteries*. All of them gave freely of their expertise and in the process enriched my understanding of these historical figures with both information and perspective.

The list of these contributors is long and includes: In the case of Tutankhamun: Irwin M. Braverman, MD (Yale University), Donald B. Redford, PhD (Pennsylvania State University), and Professor Bette Sue Masters (University of Texas San Antonio); The Buddha: Nayan Kothari, MD (St. Peter's University Hospital, New Brunswick, New Jersey); Caligula: Wayne Millan (George Washington University), Judith P. Hallett, PhD (University of Maryland), Anthony A. Barrett, PhD (University of British Columbia), and William T. Carpenter III, MD (University of Maryland); Saladin: Stuart C. Ray, MD (Johns Hopkins University); Goya: Susan Billings (Baton Rouge, Louisiana) and Gary Wormser, MD (New York Medical College); John Paul Jones: Mathew R. Weir, MD (University of Maryland), Lori L. Bogle, PhD (U.S. Naval Academy), John Wilson (U.S. Naval Academy), Cinthia Drachenberg, MD (University of Maryland), and Robert Knodell, MD (University of Maryland); Bolívar: Paul G. Auwaerter, MD (Johns Hopkins University), John Dove, MBBS (University of Edinburgh), Steven D. Munger, PhD (University of Maryland), and Adriana Naim, MD (University of Maryland); Darwin: Sidney Cohen, MD (Thomas Jefferson University) and Ruth Padel (University College

London); Jackson: Frederic T. Billings III, MD (Baton Rouge, Louisiana), Steven S. Wasserman, PhD (University of Virginia), James I. Robertson, PhD (Virginia Polytechnic and State University), Joe DuBose, MD (University of Maryland), Michael A. Flannery, PhD (University of Alabama), and Maurice S. Albin, MD (University of Alabama Birmingham); Lincoln: Thomas M. Scalea, MD (University of Maryland) and Steven L. Carson (The Abraham Lincoln Institute); Lenin: Harry Vinters, MD (University of California Los Angeles) and Lev Lurie (The St. Petersburg Classical Gimnazium, Russia); Lanza: Armando Cesari (Victoria, Australia); Roosevelt: Barron H. Lerner, MD, PhD (New York University), Virginia Lewick (F.D.R. Library), Ronald Sacher, MD (University of Cincinnati), and Maria Baer, MD (University of Maryland).

In addition to those mentioned above, I wish to thank the following people for editorial advice, literature searches, and/or artwork: Frank M. Calia, MD (University of Maryland), Larry Pitrof (University of Maryland), Morton M. Krieger, MD (University of Maryland), Virginia U. Collier, MD (Christiana Health Care System), Richard J. Behles, MLS (University of Maryland), Sabra Kurth (VA Maryland Health Care System), Seth Crawford (VA Maryland Health Care System), and Jordan Denner (VA Maryland Health Care System).

Yet will I bring one plague more upon Pharaoh and upon Egypt.

EXODUS 11:1

....

1   Mummy's Curse

WHEN THIS PATIENT became Pharaoh in ca. 1332 BCE, the Kingdom of Egypt (Fig. 1.1) (1) was nearly 2,000 years old. The pyramids at Giza had maintained silent vigil over the "gift of the Nile" for over 700 years, and 1,300 more years would elapse before the last pharaoh, Caesarion, the son of Cleopatra VII and Julius Caesar, would be murdered by order of Caesar Augustus, and the realm annexed as a property of Rome (2).

Like the pharaohs before and after him, this pharaoh presided over his land and his people as absolute monarch, overseeing every function of state, from collection of taxes and the administration of justice to the waging of war. He was only a child when Smenkhkare died and made him king. Even so, in the eyes of his people, he became an essential feature of the cosmos on ascending the throne, a derivative of the divinity of Egypt's gods, from whom his power emanated. On him, the very existence of the universe depended (3). However, until he matured into manhood, Ay, his vizier, and Horemheb, general of his northern army, advised him as co-regents (4). Both would succeed him as pharaohs.

He was a member of ancient Egypt's 18th Dynasty, 14 pharaohs who ruled Egypt during a period known as the "New Kingdom." Another 13 dynasties would direct the empire before being displaced by a Macedonian hegemony of Ptolemaic kings in the aftermath of Alexander's invasion in the 4th century BCE (5). The patient's family was one of the most powerful of all the royal houses of ancient Egypt (6). They were the ones who introduced chariot forces into Egypt's armies during a period of imperial expansion into both the upper Nile (Nubia) and Asia Minor (7). They were also the ones who succeeded in converting Syria from adversary to ally

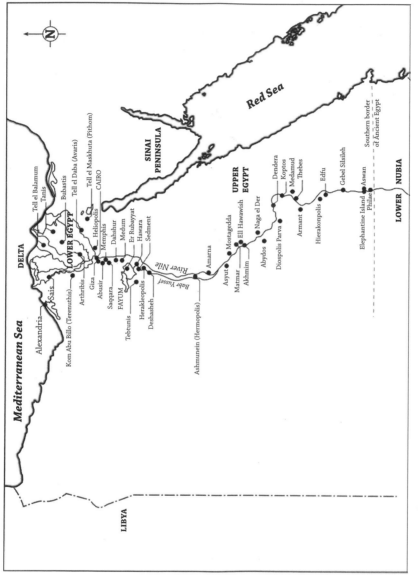

FIGURE 1.1 Ancient Upper and Lower Egypt. (Adapted from reference 1, p. 1)

in clashes with the Hittites of Anatolia (modern Turkey). Sixty years before the patient's birth, the Hittites had conquered Wilusa (Troy), only to be defeated there almost a century later by Agamemnon's Achaean forces (8). The patient was no Agamemnon and had only limited success in battling the Hittites on his northern frontier.

The patient's family presided over a time of unprecedented prosperity, stability, artistic creativity, and international prestige—at least during the dynasty's early years. Iron was introduced into Egypt during his reign, most likely by the Hittites, marking the beginning of the end of the Bronze Age, one dominated by Egypt (9). The patient's era was also a golden age of medicine (10).

Surviving medical papyri of the 18th Dynasty (11) describe a practice of medicine during this pharaoh's time that was both logical and surprisingly sophisticated, one with important lessons for our own era. Physicians then recognized the existence of the heart, liver, spleen, kidneys, ureters, and bladder and appreciated the connection between blood vessels and the heart (12). They had training manuals and practice manuals not much different from our own. They also produced one of the earliest known surgical texts, the *Edwin Smith Papyrus*. Occasionally, they invoked the gods when ministering to patients; however, probably not much more often than we do today when family members pray for favorable outcomes in desperate cases (10). Their "recitals" or incantations seem to have been prayers for skill and guidance more than attempts to invoke supernatural intervention. Although their diagnoses were frequently descriptive, merely repeating words used by patients to describe their disabilities, again, they were not terribly different from some of our own diagnoses, as for example *angina pectoris* (pain in the chest) in patients complaining of chest pain (13).

The physicians of the patient's era (and for that matter, those who preceded them for more than 1,000 years (14)) seem to have been keen, systematic, and accurate observers, who appreciated many of the same principles of diagnosis we adhere to today (15). They performed careful physical examinations using inspection, olfaction, palpation, and possibly even percussion (3,000 years before Auenbrugger reintroduced the technique into modern medical practice (16)). They had no clinical laboratory per se but nevertheless examined both the urine and the feces in their diagnostic evaluations (16). They appreciated the importance of prognosis in managing illnesses (15) and were intellectually honest—some might say more so than today's physicians—in recommending no treatment in cases deemed hopeless (10). The treatments they did administer were, on the whole, relatively simple and favored natural restorative processes involving as little injury to the patient as possible. These included amputations (17), débridement of dead tissue, incision and drainage of abscesses (18), application of poultices (such as fresh meat) and wound dressings, immobilization of injured limbs, preparation and application of splints, setting fractures, crude casts, and even simple prostheses (17, 19).

These early physicians also had an extensive pharmacopeia that included plant remedies such as acacia, anise, cassia, lotus, and wormwood, in addition to mineral remedies such as alum, copper, feldspar, sodium bicarbonate, sulfur, and possibly also arsenical compounds (20). Nearly 50 percent of the drug sources used by the ancient Egyptians remain in use today, though many are now synthesized. Nearly two thirds of the ancient compounds have been shown to be therapeutically effective (21). Many such prescriptions combined several agents, prepared according to compounding methods similar to those used in pharmacies today (22). Physicians then seemed to realize that drugs taken by mouth are apt to have more general effects than those applied to the skin. Although they had no concept of the principles of absorption or distribution, they did have a vague appreciation for the relationship between the dose of a drug and its effect (23). Long before the advent of modern antibiotics, they prevented wound infections by applying honey (a potent antibacterial agent (24)) liberally to wounds. Long before the advent of anti-inflammatory drugs, they used willow leaves, a source of salicylic acid, the key ingredient of aspirin, to reduce inflammation (25).

Like today, medical practice during the patient's era was a specialized business. According to Herodotus, in ancient Egypt, "some are physicians for the eyes, others for the head, teeth, abdomen, and for unknown diseases" (26). Herodotus did not speculate whether such specialization enhanced or hindered the quality of health care. He did, however, maintain that after the Libyans, the Egyptians were the healthiest in the world, a distinction likely related to the keen interest the state took in the health of its people, possibly even to the extent of remunerating physicians, some of whom were women, as state employees (26).

Although modern medicine generally traces its origin to the teachings of Hippocrates and his disciples (27), Greece was actually the natural successor and perpetuator of Egyptian medical practice (12). Over 1,000 years before students of Hippocrates espoused similar ideas, the ancient Egyptians entertained the idea that disease enters a person from the outside. It was the Egyptians who surmised that, in at least some cases, disease spreads through the vessels and must be eliminated in the excreta. Whereas Greek concepts of health and disease involved a belief in a delicate balance of four humors (blood, phlegm, yellow bile, and black bile), long before the Greeks formalized these concepts, the ancient Egyptians credited similar functions to circulating *st.t* (mucus), *rwt* (bile), and *whdw* (alimentary residues). Unfortunately for this patient, neither his exalted position nor the skill of his physicians could prevent his sudden death after less than a decade as pharaoh (28).

The kingdom this pharaoh inherited was disordered and demoralized as a result of his father's experiment with monotheism, during which service to all gods save Aten, the Sun Disc, had been done away with. Temples had drifted into desuetude, with loss of revenues that had sustained the daily cult and pageantry of meaningful existence for nearly 2,000 years (29). The gods, thus alienated, seemed to have withdrawn their support (30). The people had lost the will to endure and to overcome setbacks during those lean years and looked to the young king to restore their confidence and to bring back the prosperity of earlier times. The army had become unruly, the peasantry destitute, and the judiciary corrupt (31) in the wake of a ship of state that had drifted rudderless for nearly two decades (32).

When the patient became king, his first efforts (or, more appropriately, those of his regime, since he was then but 9 years old) were directed at restoring the traditional status quo—in particular, reopening temples closed by his father and rejuvenating their cults (33). Though physically weak himself, he reintroduced the traditional image of pharaoh as energetic potentate, one again imbued with the spirit of imperialism. To this end, he instructed the royal artists to produce images of him charging a fleeing enemy, and also as a sportsman king hunting in his chariot (34).

Conditions also had deteriorated on the periphery of the empire during his father's disastrous reign. The army, demoralized by years of inaction and neglect of martial virtues, was in no position to take to the field, even under a dynamic leader (35). Suppilulimas, king of the Hittites, had overrun Syria, Egypt's northern ally, and destabilized the entire plain of central Mesopotamia. The patient organized a two-pronged attack designed to drive the Hittites out of Syria. However, the campaign failed, and soon after the return of his army, the king died (36). Some have since wondered if he had been murdered. The patient was barely 18 when he entered the realm of the dead to eat the food of Osiris. Having left no heir, he was the last of the glorious Tutmosid line (37).

We know almost nothing of this patient's medical history, except that he died suddenly after ruling Egypt for less than a decade. His parents were siblings (6). He too married a sibling, a half-sister, Ankhesenamun. They produced two stillborn daughters, who were both interred with the patient. Soon after the patient died, Ankhesenamun petitioned Suppilulimas to send one of his many sons to Egypt to marry her and succeed her husband as pharaoh. However, the Hittite suitor was murdered before the plan could be consummated, and Ay, the patient's vizier, took Ankhesenamun as his wife and became pharaoh (38, 39).

The patient was slight of build and roughly 5'6" tall. He had large anterior incisors, an overbite, and a strikingly elongated head (*dolichocephaly*). He also had a cleft palate and mild scoliosis (curvature of the spine). He used a cane when walking

(6). His uncle, Smenkhkare, was also a cripple (40). In some, though not all, of the patient's images, he has breasts as large as a woman's (*gynecomastia*). Many of the images of his forefathers also exhibit gynecomastia as well as dolichocephaly.

The discovery of the patient's nearly intact tomb in 1922 by Howard Carter provided a wealth of additional clinical information without solving the mystery of this boy-king's sudden death or odd physique. The tomb contained the king's mummy, along with a profusion of priceless relics, discoveries that elevated this young king of obscure origin, and short and uneventful reign, into the most famous pharaoh of all (41). Only Champollion's decipherment of the hieroglyphic code a century earlier generated as much modern excitement as the discovery of this minor king's nearly intact tomb.

When the series of coffins encasing the pharaoh's mummy was opened in the fall of 1925, Carter and his party discovered an innermost coffin 6'1.75" in length and 2.5 to 3.5 millimeters thick of solid gold, in addition to a magnificent burnished gold mask covering the patient's head and shoulders. On the mask's forehead, wrought in massive gold, were the royal insignia of the two kingdoms over which the patient presided—the Nekhebet vulture of the upper kingdom and the Buto serpent of the lower kingdom (42).

An autopsy of the mummy begun on November 11, 1925, produced only meager results due to the age of the specimen and also because the corpse was firmly fixed to the bottom of the coffin by resinous material (unguent) that had been poured over the body after it had been placed in the coffin. The latter had to be chiseled away from beneath the limbs and the trunk before the remains could be lifted out of the coffin. Further difficulties were encountered during the examination because humidity at the time of internment, in combination with decomposition of the unguents, had generated enough heat to bring about spontaneous combustion that carbonized the linen wrappings encasing the mummy (43).

The limited findings of the postmortem examination were as follows:

> The face... [had a] remarkable structural resemblance to... Akhenaten (44)... that [the patient] was a son of Akhenaten... seems... the only possible explanation (45)... the king's head shows that, through the convention of the period, the finer contemporary representations of the king upon monuments, beyond all doubt, are accurate portraits (46)... the upper lip is slightly elevated revealing... large central incisor teeth... On the left cheek, just in front of the lobe of the ear, is a rounded depression, the skin filling it, resembling a scab... The head when fully uncovered was seen to be very broad and flat topped (platycephalic) with markedly projecting occipital region [the posterior region]... which is of a very uncommon type... like that

of…Akhenaten. The skull cavity was empty except for some resinous material which had been introduced through the nose…[was] now of rock-like
hardness…There was no pubic hair visible…but the phallus had been drawn
forward…the lower end of the femur was thus exposed, showing the epi-
physis [the growth plate]…to be separate from the shaft and freely movable
[indicating an age of 18–19 years]…The limbs appeared very shrunken and
attenuated…evident that [the patient] must have been of slight build and
perhaps not fully grown at the time of his death…the examination afforded
no clue to the cause of his early death. (47)

In 1968, examination of x-rays of the patient's skull by R. G. Harrison of the University
of Liverpool revealed a small piece of bone inside the cranial cavity, thought to repre-
sent either a piece of ethmoid bone dislodged when an instrument had been inserted
through the nose during the embalming process or, possibly, a bone fragment that
had fused with the overlying skull during healing of a depressed skull fracture (48).
The latter interpretation raised the possibility of a brain hemorrhage caused by a
blow to the head from a blunt instrument or fall. Given the patient's sudden demise
and hasty burial and the troubled times in which he lived, murder surfaced as a possible cause of death (orchestrated by his successors Ay and Horemheb, for example,
or even Ankhesenamun). However, on re-examination of the x-rays in 2003, radiolo-
gists at the Children's Medical Center of the University of Utah concluded that the
bone fragment and questionable hemorrhage represented nothing more than post-
mortem artifacts resulting from the mummification process and/or trauma inflicted
during the 1925 autopsy (49). The cause of death remained unanswered.

For nearly 2,000 years those seeking to unlock this and countless other mysteries
of ancient Egypt relied solely on guesswork and hypothesis (50). This all changed
in 1799 with the discovery by Napoleon's soldiers of a slab of black basalt 3'10"
high buried in the sand near the Delta village of Rosetta (now Rashid) (51, 52).
Etched onto the surface of this "Rosetta stone" was a commemorative decree in
three scripts—hieroglyphs, Greek, and Demotic (ancient Egyptian)—which in
1822 finally enabled Jean-François Champollion to decipher the meaning of hieroglyphs, ancient Egypt's recorded language for more than 3,000 years. Initially,
scholars thought the characters were symbolic in nature and couldn't break the
code of the long-forgotten script. Only when Champollion and others recognized
that they were actually phonetic representations was the veil finally lifted from the
records of ancient Egypt. After the code was broken, the pharaohs could be identified by name and their deeds scrutinized. Only then was it possible to pronounce
the two names by which this pharaoh was known—Tutankhaten ("Living image of
Aten"), Tutankhamun ("Living image of Amun")…today's King Tut.

Champollion's work gave us the name of the boy-king but not the reason for his untimely death. It took another autopsy performed in 2010 to begin to unravel that mystery. This one, conducted under the auspices of the Egyptian Supreme Council of Antiquities, involved detailed anthropological, radiological, and genetic studies of Tutankhamun and 10 other royal mummies (6). Genetic tests performed on DNA extracted from Tut's bones detected evidence of infection with two different strains of the malaria parasite, *Plasmodium falciparum*. Tests for bubonic plague, tuberculosis, leprosy, and leishmaniasis (a parasitic infection transmitted by sand flies) were negative. Positive tests for *P. falciparum* obtained in three of the other mummies proved that malaria was endemic in Egypt at the time of Tutankhamun.

Falciparum malaria is the deadliest form of malaria (53). However, in endemic areas, children are repeatedly infected with the parasite and bear the main burden of life-threatening disease. Those who survive their initial infection develop immunity to the parasite, protecting them from clinical symptoms (and death) when reinfected. Therefore, if malaria had killed Tutankhamun, more than likely it would have done so during the course of his initial infection, before he had developed antibodies against the parasite. By the time he had reached the age of 18 and had been infected at least twice, he should have had enough immunity to have survived yet another bout of falciparum malaria—that is, unless he had some other medical problem that had weakened his resistance over time. Moreover, if he had red blood cells containing an abnormal hemoglobin (such as the one responsible for sickle cell anemia), as has been suggested by Timmann (54), his erythrocytes (red blood cells) would have been resistant to invasion by falciparum malaria. If not malaria, what could have killed him?

In the studies conducted by the Supreme Council of Antiquities investigators, several other abnormalities were detected in the boy-king's mummy, perhaps relevant to the question of the cause of his death. Computed axial tomography (CAT scan) revealed an arch of the right foot that was abnormally low (flat-footed), whereas the arch of the left foot was slightly higher than normal. Several of the bones of the left foot were defective, and the forefoot was inwardly rotated, akin to a club foot deformity. There was also a fractured leg (possibly sustained during a military skirmish or hunting expedition (37)), a cleft palate, and mild curvature of the spine (kyphoscoliosis).

Construction of a five-generation pedigree of Tut's immediate lineage using genetic fingerprinting provided a probable explanation for these deformities, many of which were shared by Tutankhamun's ancestors. The analysis confirmed what many had long suspected—the mummy discovered in tomb KV 55 (tomb #55 in the Valley of the Kings) was that of the son of Amenhotep III (Tut's grandfather) and almost certainly Akhenaten. More important, further genetic fingerprinting identified the KV55 mummy as Tutankhamun's father and another mummy, KV35YL, the sister of KV55, as his mother. Thus, Tutankhamun, husband to his own half-sister, was the offspring of a brother–sister union and a product of generations of inbreeding that might well have been responsible for not just his skeletal anomalies but possibly also other undetected anomalies involving his vital organs (see below).

In 1980, Dr. Bernadine Paulshock first called attention to evidence of familial gynecomastia in the 18th-Dynasty pharaohs after viewing a statue of Tutankhamun with such well-defined breasts that one would have thought it was the image of a young woman were it not for the pharaonic headgear (Fig. 1.2)

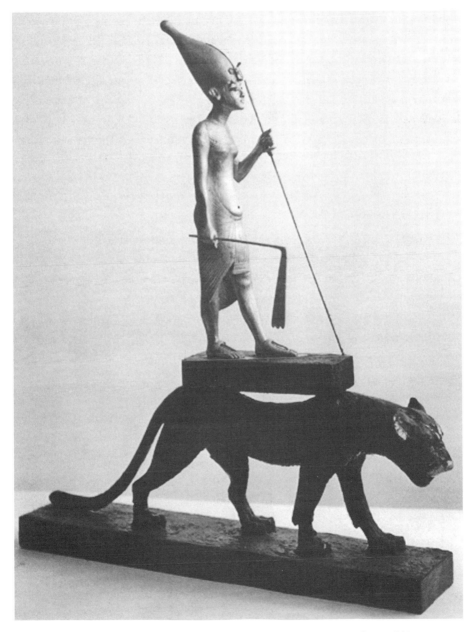

FIGURE 1.2 Statue of tutankhamun with pronounced gynecomastia on a leopard (Cairo Museum No. 60714).

(55). Smenkhkare, Tut's uncle (possibly his brother) and immediate predecessor, was also depicted with gynecomastia so pronounced that a relief of him in the Berlin Museum was for a long time thought to be a portrait of Nefertiti. Subsequent systematic examination of images of Tutankhamun and his forefathers revealed evidence of not only gynecomastia in each of the Tutmosid pharaohs of the 18th Dynasty (Tut's patrilineal line) but also several instances of cranial abnormalities similar to Tutankhamun's (Table 1.1) (56). Images of Akhenaten's young daughters show both marked dolichocephaly and isosexual precocity (premature breast and hip development) (Fig. 1.3). Gynecomastia is both striking and widespread among images of the Tutmosid pharaohs. However, it is inconsistently represented, being present in some but not all of their images. Moreover, gynecomastia is present in images of commoners as well as the pharaohs of other dynasties (57), though not nearly as often as in images of the Tutmosids, raising the possibility that the abnormality is

TABLE 1.1

Images Depicting Endocrine and Cranial Abnormalities in the Principal Rulers of Egypt's 18th Dynasty*

Ruler	Gynecomastia	Cranial Abnormality
Amosis	No data**	Absent
Amenophis I	Absent	Absent
Thutmose I†	Present	Present
Thutmose II	Absent	Present
Queen Hatshepsut	Not applicable	Present
Thutmose III	No data**	Present
Amenophis II	Present	No data**
Thutmose IV	Present	Present
Amenophis III	Present	Present
Amenophis IV/Akhenaten	Present	Present
Smenkhkare	Present	Present
Tutankhamun†	Present	Present
Aye	Absent	Absent
Horemheb	Absent	Absent

* Adapted from Braverman et al. (reference 56).

** The presence or absence of cranial or endocrine abnormality in any statuary, painting, mummy, or relief.

† Patrilineal line of Tutankhamun begins with Thutmose I and ends with Tutankhamun.

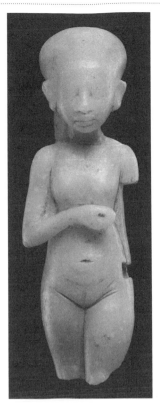

FIGURE 1.3 Alabaster statuette of one of Akhenaten's daughters (the patient's half-sister) at 3 to 5 years of age, exhibiting an elongated head, well-developed breasts, and prominent hips. (Reproduced with permission from Museum für Kunst und Gewerbe Hamburg: Abbeldung; 1965: Abbildung 53, Katalog Nr. 23)

symbolic rather than realistic. However, isosexual precocity is seen only in the images of Akhenaten's daughters. If the gynecomastia and isosexual precocity were actual physical traits of the 18th Dynasty (rather than symbolic representations), they could be explained only by an inherited disorder of estrogen metabolism—specifically, the aromatase excess syndrome.

Aromatase (also called "estrogen synthetase") is an enzyme that converts male hormones, such as testosterone, into estrogenic, female hormones (56). These conversions occur normally and are critical to the physiological transformations that occur during puberty. However, in patients with aromatase excess syndrome, mutations in the genes responsible for aromatase synthesis cause the enzyme (and hence estrogenic hormones) to be produced in such abnormally high amounts that affected males develop gynecomastia and affected females precocious sexual characteristics.

The strange elongated skulls of members of the 18th Dynasty (58) also are best explained by a defective gene, passed from one generation to the next in a genetic code riddled with abnormal genes. In this case, the defective gene is one of several responsible for fusion of the various bony plates that unite to form the rigid skull of the adult (Fig. 1.4). There are five such plates (or bones): the frontal bone (which forms the forehead), the parietal bone (the upper half of the side of the skull), the temporal bone (the lower half of the side of the skull), the sphenoid bone (the anterior temple region), and the occipital bone (the back of the skull). Narrow spaces (or joints), called *sutures*, separate these bones and enable the immature skull to expand as the brain grows. Once the brain is fully grown, the sutures fuse to form the rigid bony container that is the adult skull.

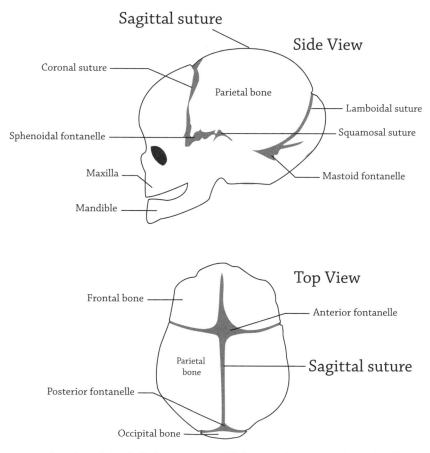

FIGURE 1.4 Drawing of the skull of a newborn child showing the various plates that fuse to form the adult skull and the location of the sagittal suture.

If the sutures fuse too early, the immature brain is trapped within a noncompliant container and becomes progressively compressed as it attempts to grow. Pressure increases within the cranium, which if not relieved leads to blindness and mental retardation. If some, but not all, of the bony plates of the immature skull fuse prematurely, the brain is able to grow, but only in the direction of those plates that have not yet fused. In cases of dolichocephaly, the suture separating the two parietal plates (the sagittal suture) fuses prematurely, preventing the uppermost part of the brain from expanding laterally and forcing it to grow downward, as well as anteriorly and posteriorly in the direction of plates not yet fused. This particular disorder, known as craniosynostosis of the sagittal suture (i.e., premature fusion of the midline suture), is the most common inherited craniosynostosis responsible for dolichocephaly. It produces an abnormally elongated head with bulging temples (as in Fig. 1.3) but does not cause increased intracranial pressure or mental retardation. Several abnormal genes responsible for the disorder have been identified. Unfortunately, tests for these genes were not performed on any of the mummies examined by the Supreme Council of Antiquities investigators.

These various abnormalities, while disfiguring, would not likely have been responsible for Tutankhamun's death, nor would they have impaired his capacity to survive falciparum malaria. However, if he had had yet other genetic defects, ones affecting vital organs such as his heart, blood, or kidney, these defects combined with a bout of malaria or a fractured leg might have created enough of a strain on his frail constitution to have been fatal.

The odds against Tutankhamun's having had four genetic defects (club foot, cleft palate, aromatase excess syndrome, and cranial synostosis), much less five or more genetic defects, would seem to be improbably high. Given the results of his recent radiological examination, it seems clear that he had a club foot, as well as a cleft palate. However, his gynecomastia and dolichocephaly, like those of other pharaohs in his patrilineal line, are portrayed inconsistently and might have been symbolic rather than real. Nevertheless, Tutankhamun was a product of a heavily inbred extended family (59), which placed him at considerable risk of such defects. Could inbreeding have resulted in five or more genetic disorders?

While we have substantial information on the consequences of inbreeding involving first cousins, we have only scant information about the offsprings of first-degree relatives (brother–sister, father–daughter) and virtually none on repeated first-degree unions in extended families. Even so, it is clear that inbreeding increases the likelihood of both infant mortality and congenital birth defects (60, 61) and that as the amount of inbreeding increases, so do the frequency and the complexity of congenital malformations (62). This is because inbreeding increases the chance that a fertilized egg will possess two copies of deleterious recessive alleles (i.e., genes or groups of genes responsible for defects only when present in two copies, one from the mother and another from the father) (60, 63). Because most such alleles are rare, it is unlikely that two parents will both be carriers of the same deleterious allele. However, because close relatives share a great many alleles (good as well as bad), the probability that a rare deleterious allele present in a common ancestor will be inherited from two closely related parents increases markedly.

One of the very few reports dealing with children born of incestuous unions (father–daughter, brother–sister) was published by Baird and McGillivray in 1982 (64). It described the status of 21 such children. Two died suddenly in the first months of life. Three had minor physical abnormalities. Of the remainder, 9 (43 percent) had serious physical defects that were thought to be congenital in origin. Most of the children had multiple malformations. One had five, all of which were apparent at 1 year of age: ear pits, atrial septal defect (a congenital heart defect), bilateral vertical talus ("rocker bottom" feet), moderate mental retardation, and subluxated (congenitally dislocated) hips. Because many of the other children were quite young when evaluated, the authors speculated that further congenital problems would likely be identified as they grew older. In view of these observations and given Tutankhamun's heavily inbred extended family, the odds of his having five or more congenital abnormalities, some of which involved vital organs, would have been high.

On November 26, 1922, George Edward Stanhope Molyneux Herbert, fifth Earl of Carnarvon (Fig. 1.5), entered Tutankhamun's tomb, as was his right and reward for providing the financial support that made the tomb's discovery possible. Five months later, he was dead, killed by an attack of erysipelas complicated by pneumonia. When another member of the team of 24 people present when the tomb was opened suffered a fatal stroke, many began to wonder if a "mummy's curse" was responsible for not just those two deaths but also more to come (65). Although early press reports and subsequent horror movies perpetuated the idea that desecrators of Tut's tomb were doomed, a retrospective cohort study published in 2002 of 44 Westerners potentially exposed to the same curse found no association between exposure to the tomb and death. Thus, if a curse existed, its victims would not appear to have been the desecrators of the king's tomb. But was there a "curse"? And if so, who were its victims, and what was its source?

Given the foregoing information, it is difficult to deny the existence of a curse, one imposed by Min, ancient Egypt's god of fertility, on the entire clan of Tutmosids. They were cursed for having committed repeated sins of incest.

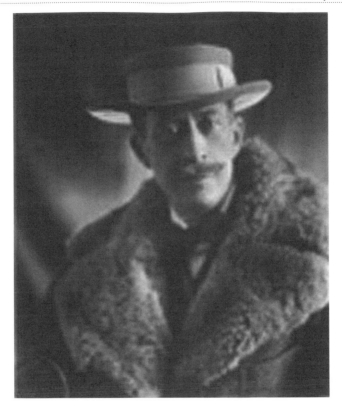

FIGURE 1.5 Lord Carnarvon. The chief financial backer of Howard Carter's excavations, which led to the discovery of Tutankhamun's tomb.

Tutankhamun, in particular, was cursed for having been born a child of incest and a descendent of this highly inbred extended family. The evil fortunes visited upon him by the curse included multiple congenital abnormalities, two stillborn daughters, and his own death before he could leave his imprint as earthly God King on a 5,000-year-old kingdom.

References

1. Russmann ER. *Eternal Egypt. Masterworks of Ancient Art from the British Museum*. Berkeley: University of California Press, 2001:15.

2. Aldred C. *Akhenaten. King of Egypt*. London: Thames & Hudson, 1988:9.

3. Silverman DP. *Ancient Egypt*. New York: Oxford University Press, 1997:106.

4. Op. cit. Aldred, p. 295).

5. Ibid., p. 20.

6. Hawass Z, Gad YZ, Ismail S, et al. Ancestry and pathology in King Tutankhamun's family. *JAMA* 2010;303:638–647.

7. Op. cit. Aldred, p. 96.

8. Staecker H, Easton D, Mackowiak PA. The last myrmidon. The life, legacy, and fatal ear disorder of Heinrich Schliemann. *The Pharos* 2006;69:12–18.

9. Carter H. *The Tomb of Tutankhamen*. Portland: Excalibur Books, 1972:154.

10. Leake CD. *The Old Egyptian Medical Papyri*. Lawrence: University of Kansas Press, 1952:35–36.

11. Mackowiak PA. *Post Mortem. Solving History's Great Medical Mysteries*. Philadelphia: ACP Press, 2007:20–21.

12. Ghalioungui P. *Magic and Medical Science in Ancient Egypt*. London: Hodder and Stoughton, 1963.

13. Op. cit. Leake, p. 10.

14. Ibid., p. 13.

15. Ibid., pp. 16–17.

16. Op. cit. Ghalioungui, pp. 115–117.

17. Nerlich AG, Zink A, Szeimies U, Hagedorn JG. Ancient Egyptian prosthesis of the big toe. *Lancet* 2000;356:2176–2179.

18. Op. cit. Leake, p. 61.

19. Ibid., pp. 39–40.

20. Op. cit. Leake, pp. 41–42.

21. David R. The art of healing in ancient Egypt: a scientific reappraisal. *Lancet* 2008;372:1802–1803.

22. Op. cit. Leake, p. 45.

23. Ibid., p. 30.

24. Mackowiak PA. Brief history of antipyretic therapy. *Clin Infect Dis* 2000;31 (Suppl 5):S154–156.

25. Kwakman PHS, Van den Akker JPC, Guclu A, et al. Medical-grade honey kills antibiotic-resistant bacteria in vitro and eradicates skin colonization. *Clin Infect Dis* 2008;46:1677–1682.

26. Op. cit. Ghalioungui, p. 18.

27. Op. cit. (Mackowiak), pp. 39–43.

28. Op. cit. (Silverman), p. 109.

29. Redford DB. *Akhenaten. The Heretic King*. Princeton University Press. Princeton: 1984:169–70.

30. Op. cit. Aldred, p. 294.

31. Op. cit. Redford, p. 224.

32. Ibid., p. 205.

33. Ibid., p. 208.

34. Ibid., p. 211.

35. Op. cit. Aldred, p. 283.

36. Op. cit. Redford, pp. 212–215.

37. Op. cit. Aldred, p. 297.

38. Ibid., p. 298.

39. Op. cit. Redford, pp. 216–221.

40. Op. cit. Aldred, p. 250.

41. Ibid., p. 108.

42. Op. cit. Carter, pp. 126–130.

43. Ibid., pp. 140–141.

44. Ibid., p. 144.

45. Ibid., p. 145.

46. Ibid., p. 146.

47. Ibid., pp. 226–231.

48. Harrison RG. Post mortem on two pharaohs: was Tutankhamen's skull fractured? *Buried History* 1971;4:114–129.

49. Boyer RS, Rodin EA, Grey TC, Connolly RC. The skull and cervical spine radiographs of Tutankhamen: a critical appraisal. *Am J Neuroradiol* 2003;24:1142–1147.

50. Op. cit. Silverman, p. 6.

51. Ibid., pp. 230–231.

52. Op. cit. Russmann, p. 47.

53. Op. cit. Mackowiak, pp. 70–72.

54. Timmann C. King Tutankhamun's family and demise [letter]. *JAMA* 2010;303:2473.

55. Paulshock BZ. Tutankhamun and his brothers. Familial gynecomastia in the eighteenth dynasty. *JAMA* 1980;244:160–164.

56. Braverman IM, Redford DB, Mackowiak PA. Akhenaten and the strange physiques of Egypt's 18th dynasty. *Ann Intern Med* 2009;150:556–561.

57. Op. cit. Russmann, p. 34.

58. Op. cit. Aldred, p. 76.

59. Op. cit. Redford, p. 193.

60. Bittles AH, Neel JV. The costs of human inbreeding and their implications for variations at the DNA level. *Nature Genet* 1994;8:117–121.

61. Seemanova E. A study of children of incestuous matings. *Human Heredity* 1971;21:108–128.

62. Schull WJ. Empirical risks in consanguineous marriages: sex ratio, malformations, and viability. *Am J Hum Genet* 1958;10:294–343.

63. Livingstone FB. Genetics, ecology and the origins of incest and exogamy. *Current Anthropology* 1969;10:45–62.

64. Baird PA, McGillivray. Children of incest. *J Pediatr* 1982;101:354–357.

65. Nelson MR. The mummy's curse: historical cohort study. *Br Med J* 2002;325:1482–484.

2   Last Repast

THIS PATIENT IS revered for having fomented a religious revolution against the dominant evils of Brahmanism. He rejected the caste system, bloody sacrifices, and the authority of the Vedas. He promoted moral enlightenment through self-less endeavor over trust in rituals. His gospel continues to resonate with millions throughout the world even today, more than 2,000 years after his death. It advocates a comprehensive love for all creatures intertwined with a belief in reincarnation. It stresses a "Middle Way" between a life of indulgence and one of harsh austerity in developing understanding in religious as well as secular matters, through personal experience (1).

The patient was born in the Terai lowlands of India, near the foothills of the Himalayas, during the 6th century BCE. His people were members of the Gotama clan of the Sakya tribe. Tradition has it that his family belonged to the second of the four Indian castes—the aristocratic warrior caste known as the *khattiyas*. However, some scholars doubt that a caste system actually existed among the Sakya during the patient's day (2).

Only fragments of the patient's life were recorded for posterity. In fact, no attempt was made to piece together the details of his life story into a continuous narrative until over 400 years after his death. Moreover, the first narrative as well as other later versions are embellished with fanciful details that make it difficult to separate fact from legend (2, 3). Nevertheless, certain key elements of the patient's life and medical history are reasonably well established.

His family was apparently well-to-do. His father, Suddhodana ("Pure Rice"), might even have been a nobleman. Not much else is known of him or of the patient's mother, Maya ("Illusion"). She died of unknown cause just 7 days after the patient's birth, leaving the baby boy to be raised by her sister, Pājapatī, who became Suddhodana's second wife (2).

The patient reportedly grew up in a luxurious environment, secluded within the walls of his father's three palaces, one for each of the three seasons of the Indian year. He wore fine garments and was surrounded by musicians and pampered by a host of attendants. Even so, he emerged not as a spoiled child, but one who was considerate and also precocious, with a keen intelligence and latent psychic powers (2).

He is reported to have been extraordinarily gifted both mentally and physically, excelling in subjects and activities as diverse as mathematics and wrestling, poetry and archery, and music and driving a chariot. He had curly blue-black hair with a snow-white tuft in the middle of his brow, a broad smooth forehead, and a prominent lump jutting out of the front of his skull. His eyes were black, his teeth perfectly white and 40 in number. His chest and shoulders were broad and his skin soft and golden. His arms reached to his knees when he stood erect. His fingers and toes were long and webbed, his nails rounded. He had a powerful gait with a tendency to veer to the right when he walked (4). On looking backwards, he would turn his whole body "as an elephant does" (5).

Although palace life was comfortable, the patient yearned for a deeper, more spiritually satisfying existence. During repeated excursions outside the confines of his father's palaces, he encountered first the ravages of old age, then disease and death, and finally had a spiritual awakening under the influence of a religious almsman (samana). Shortly thereafter, he decided to leave forever his father's palaces and his sleeping wife and child in search of spiritual enlightenment as a homeless mendicant (2).

His first teacher, a man named Ālāra Kālāma, taught him a meditational technique that enabled him to abide in a profound trance-like state known as the "sphere of nothingness." The experience was serene and blissful but not the complete, permanent transformation he sought. He encountered another teacher, Uddaka Rāmaputta, who introduced him to a more advanced meditational technique, which transported him to a mental sphere of neither perception nor non-perception, but an even more sublime state of mind in which consciousness itself seemed to disappear. This technique too was pleasing but did not produce the spiritual transformation the patient sought (2).

After these experiments with meditation, he turned to extreme austerity as a means of subduing his appetites and passions. First, he practiced breath control, holding his breath for longer and longer periods of time. Then he resorted to self-mortification through an extreme fast in his quest for perfect enlightenment (*sambodhi*) (2). His fast lasted 6 years, during which time he consumed as little as one spoonful of bean soup a day (2)—according to one account, surely apocryphal, a single juniper berry, a single sesame seed, and a single grain of rice (6). He became increasingly emaciated and weak. By the time he ended the fast, his "rib cage was like an old stable with its sides caved in; [his] head withered until it looked old and wrinkled and dry;" his eyeballs were sunken, and he had difficulty seeing. When he placed his hand on his abdomen he could feel his spine; when he tried to stand, he fell backwards; his beautiful clear skin turned as black as the color of the madgura fish; and "all the hairs came away from his body." Before he ended the fast, he was so debilitated mentally and physically that "when the sun fell on him, he did not move into the shade, and from the shade he did not move into the sun. He did not seek refuge from the wind, sun, or rain; he did not chase away horseflies, mosquitoes, or snakes. He did not excrete urine or excrement or spittle or nasal secretions ... [he became] so weak, so feeble and thin that when they put grass and cotton in the openings of his ears, it came out through his nostrils" (6).

In time, the patient abandoned this experiment too and came to realize that the most productive course to enlightenment was a "middle way" in which appetites were neither denied nor indulged. Acting on this principle, he began to take food and returned to the practice of meditation. One night, seated beneath the Bodhi tree, he finally attained the complete state of awakening he had sought for so long. Finally, he was able to look back through his previous existences with a clairvoyant power that allowed him to see the death and rebirth of all types of beings in the universe according to their good and bad deeds. His craving and ignorance were rooted out once and forever. He had attained nirvana and put an end to rebirth. He had become the *Tathāgata* (one who has attained what is really so). He spent the remainder of his days traveling on foot through the towns and villages of northeast India teaching people of diverse religious, social, and economic backgrounds how they too might find nirvana (2).

Only fragments of the patient's medical history are available for analysis. At some time during midlife, he was given a purgative of "lotuses mixed with various medicines" by his personal physician, Jivaka Komarabhacca (see below), for "a disturbance of the humours of his body." A Sanskrit Tibetan version of the illness characterized it as "chills and a runny nose," a Chinese version as "cold sweats." Nothing more is known of its nature. On another occasion, Jivaka treated him for a backache the physician attributed to "an affliction of the wind" (7).

As far as we know, the patient's health was otherwise robust until he reached the end of his eighth decade. He was preaching in far northeast India in the vicinity of Vaiśāli (Devanagari) when he became ill. It was the rainy season. He confided in his faithful disciple of 30 years, Ânanda: "I ... am now grown old, and full of years; my journey is drawing to its close; I have reached my sum of days; I am turning eighty years of age; and just as a worn-out cart, Ânanda, can only with much additional care be made to move along; so methinks [my] body...can only be kept going with much additional care." At this time there fell upon him a dire sickness with pains so intense, his followers feared he might die. Some ancient sources attributed the attack to a chronic gastric upset, possibly dysentery (3), but the precise details of the attack are long forgotten. Though initially his pain was extreme, the patient bore it without complaint and by an extraordinary effort of will bent the sickness down and maintained his hold on life until the time he had fixed for his death (exactly 3 months from then) was at hand. The location of his pain is not recorded, nor is it known if he had had attacks of a similar nature prior to this one (8).

During the ensuing 3 months, he traveled 140 km on foot to Pāvā, a village near Kusinārā in northern Bihar where the *mahāparinirvāna* ("the Great Decease/Final Extinction") was scheduled to take place (3). He continued to promote his doctrine as he traveled. Whether he had recurrences of the above symptoms during this time is not recorded.

When he arrived in Pāvā, Cunda, a lowly metalworker, offered him shelter and began preparing the next day's meal for the patient and his disciples. The meal consisted of sweet rice, cakes, and a quantity of *sūkara-maddava* (variously translated as dried boar's flesh, "pig's delight," soft rice in a broth of milk, curd, buttermilk, butter, and ghee, and an elixir). Early the next morning, as Cunda made ready to serve his meal, the patient instructed him to serve the sweet rice and cakes to his disciples and the *sūkara-maddava* to him alone, which he claimed only he could digest. He then said to the metalworker: "Whatever *sūkara-maddava*, Cunda, is left over to you, that bury in a hole" (9).

"As soon as he had eaten Cunda's food...there fell upon [the patient] a dire sickness, the disease of dysentery, and sharp pain came upon him, even unto death. But [he], mindful and self-possessed, bore it without complaint...then after nature was relieved...announced...I am going to Kusinārā." However, he soon wearied and had to rest. He was thirsty and asked for water three times before Ânanda found some in a nearby stream clear enough to drink. A thunderstorm erupted just as a large caravan of carts roared through the vicinity. Though "conscious and awake, [the patient] neither saw, nor heard the sound of the...carts passing by, one after the other, and each close to him ...nor the sound when the falling rain went on beating and splashing, and the lightning was flashing forth, and the thunderbolts were crashing" (10). Ânanda noticed that the patient's color had become so "exceedingly bright, white, shining, and beautiful above all expression," the gold robe he was wearing seemed to have lost its luster.

The patient walked to a nearby river where he bathed and drank. He was exhausted and lay down on his right side between two Sâla trees with one foot resting on the other (12). "Then the Blessed One entered into the first stage of deep meditation. And rising out of the first stage he passed into the second. And rising out of the second he passed into the third. And rising out of the third he passed into the fourth. And rising out of the fourth stage of deep meditation he entered into the state of mind to which the infinity of space is alone present" (13). Siddhartha Gotama, the Buddha (Fig. 2.1), achieved *mahāparinirvāna* on precisely the day he had predicted he would die 3 months earlier.

The teachings of the Buddha and what little information there is concerning his life and medical history are recorded in various collections of scripture know as canons. These were preserved by means of communal chanting until the middle of the 1st century BCE, approximately 400 years after the Buddha's death, when Sri Lankan monks finally committed them to writing in the Pali Canon, so named because it is written in Pali, an extinct vernacular similar to that spoken by the Buddha (2). Five other master recensions of his life were produced in later centuries, four in Chinese and one in Sanskrit (3). They differ one from another in details of both the Buddha's life and his teachings. As the oldest narrative, the Pali Canon is widely accepted as the most authoritative (7) and is the one on which the preceding case summary is based.

Because parables, metaphors, and similes form such an important part of the Buddhist canons, it is difficult to know where fact ends and myth begins in the *Tathāgata*'s life story. Nevertheless, with regard to his terminal illness, several elements seem certain. The illness began during India's rainy season. It struck suddenly and ferociously when old age, the harbor of all ills, was already weighing heavily on the Buddha. It remitted, possibly through an extraordinary effort of will on the Buddha's part, only to recur in even greater intensity 3 months later following a meal of uncertain composition. Whether there were other attacks of the same disorder is not known, nor is it known whether the first attack, like the final one, followed a meal. Although excruciating pain was the Buddha's predominant symptom, its location is not recorded. Nevertheless, because the pain was accompanied by dysentery (bloody diarrhea) and because it was not accompanied by vomiting, it was almost certainly abdominal in location, and the source of the problem was likely the lower, rather than the upper, intestine, since vomiting is typical of disorders of the latter.

The Buddha lived to be 80, no doubt because of an uncommonly robust constitution. He was also the beneficiary of surprisingly sophisticated medical care provided by his personal physician, Jivaka Komarabhacca, which might also have contributed to his longevity.

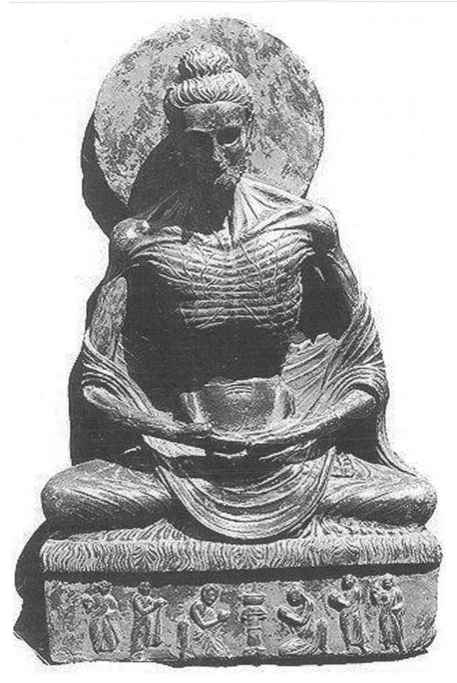

FIGURE 2.1 Second-century BCE sculpture of the starving Buddha (Lahore Museum, Lahore, Pakistan).

Jivaka received his medical training in Taxila, a city in northwest India (now northeast Pakistan) no longer in existence. He provided free medical care for the Buddha and his monks. He practiced traditional Ayurvedic medicine, a holistic form of medical care that flourishes throughout the Indian subcontinent to this day. It has its origins in ancient Hindu texts (the Vedas) written around 3000 BCE, which promote a comprehensive code of living and behavior intended to produce physical as well as spiritual well-being. The early Ayurvedic literature relates illness to supernatural influences. Initially, treatments consisted mainly of prayers and incantations. However, practical methods were also used to improve hygiene and to advance health. Plants and animal products were sometimes used to relieve symptoms (7).

By the 6th century BCE, Ayurvedic physicians such as Jivaka were practicing a form of medicine as sophisticated as that being practiced in classical Greece, if not more so. Like Hippocratic physicians, they had a high level of anatomical knowledge, a humoral theory of pathophysiology involving wind, phlegm, and bile, an empirical approach to diagnosis, and an extensive pharmacopoeia. Their surgical practice was unrivalled. It featured 122 different surgical instruments and an astonishingly advanced array of operations that included rhinoplasty, hernia repair, trephination (creating bur holes in the skull), and laparotomy (abdominal surgery). Jivaka's own practice is illustrative. Among six of his case summaries reported in the Mahavagga Sūtra, one involved incision and drainage of an abscess of the head, and another, surgical correction of a posttraumatic intestinal volvulus (i.e., unraveling a twisted segment of bowel) through an abdominal incision. A third case, mentioned above, involved the treatment of the Buddha for "a disturbance of the humours of the body" with repeated doses of a purgative (7).

Eventually, old age overtook the Buddha, and neither his sturdy constitution nor Jivaka's expert medical care could prevent the physical decay that was its companion. Old age is an incurable disease. Body parts eventually wear out and are no longer capable of sustaining life. Nevertheless, "old age" is an ambiguous diagnosis. Today, we insist on a more specific cause of death, one that explains death in terms of a particular anatomical, physiological, or molecular catastrophe. Could the Buddha's fasting some half a lifetime earlier have set in motion the process that culminated in his particular medical catastrophe?

Given the duration and the magnitude of the Buddha's fast, and the adverse physiological consequences of starvation, it is remarkable that he survived the experience, much less lived to the ripe old age of 80. During the first several days of starvation, the body depletes its stores of glycogen (carbohydrate) in the liver and muscle. This is associated with progressive weight loss and increased urinary excretion of sodium. When glycogen stores are exhausted after 10 to 14 days, muscle begins to break down, releasing amino acids (protein's building blocks), which replace glycogen as the starving body's primary energy source. Eventually, as a result of the progressive loss of protein from skeletal as well as cardiac muscle, amino acids diminish to only 10 percent of the energy source and are replaced by ketones coming from the breakdown of fatty acids contained in adipose tissue (14).

Initially, dizziness and lightheadedness, due in part to orthostatic hypotension (a drop in blood pressure on standing), are the most disabling symptoms of starvation. For this reason, starving persons like the Buddha learn to stand up slowly. By the third week of extreme fasting, hypotension and bradycardia (low pulse rate) are so profound that patients are unable to stand without assistance. Thyroid function decreases as the body modulates its metabolism in an effort to conserve energy. This leads to additional weakness along with cold intolerance. Abdominal pain develops in many patients for unknown reasons (14).

Dehydration is the most lethal complication of starvation. As illustrated by victims of Germany's concentration camps during World War II, people can survive for many months to years under near-total starvation if adequately hydrated. In the absence of water, however, death occurs in less than a fortnight (15). Thus, although not specifically stated in the Pali Canon, the Buddha's intake of water during his fast likely was restricted only marginally, if at all.

During the later phases of starvation, the consequences of vitamin deficiencies are pronounced. In the Buddha's case, his beautiful clear complexion turning as black as "the color of the madgura fish," his difficulty seeing, his hair falling out, and his extreme lethargy were as much a consequence of deficiencies of vitamins such as niacin, thiamine, and vitamins A and C as of his hypoactive thyroid and protein malnutrition. That he survived his fast is nothing short of miraculous. More often than not, death is the outcome of such prolonged starvation. When the body mass index (BMI), a standardized ratio of weight to height, falls below half of normal, vital organs such as the liver and heart begin to fail (15). Given the description of the extent of the Buddha's emaciation during the depths of his fast, his BMI would have been well below half of normal, and, hence, his risk of vital organ failure and death extreme. However, the claim that his emaciation was so pronounced that when grass was put in his ear, it came out of his nostrils seems so unlikely that it raises concern about the validity of other aspects of the Pali text. In fact, the inner ear is connected to the nasal cavity (the nasopharynx) via the Eustachian tube (Fig. 2.2). Thus, this detail of the account of the Buddha's fast is possible, and if true, indicates that the Tathāgata had a perforated ear drum on the side in which the straw was inserted.

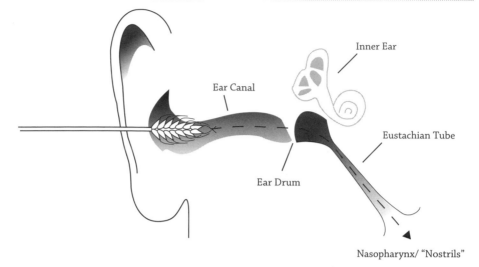

FIGURE 2.2 Anatomy of the ear, showing how grass inserted into the ear canal might find its way through a perforated ear drum to the "nostrils" via the Eustachian tube.

Once the Buddha's fast was over, he was not immediately out of danger. Following starvation, refeeding carries its own risks. Carbohydrates are especially dangerous because they divert limited stores of thiamine (vitamin B1) away from the brain and the heart into glucose metabolism. This can result in potentially fatal, acute cardiac failure (wet beriberi) and brain dysfunction (Wernicke's encephalopathy) (14). There are also long-term adverse effects of starvation on the arteries. Twenty-five years after the siege of Leningrad by Hitler's army, men surviving the nearly 3 years of famine exhibited higher blood pressures and more body fat, and were significantly more likely to die of a heart attack or a stroke than men who hadn't experienced such starvation (16).

According to the Pali Canon, "when the Buddha looked backwards, he would turn his whole body around as an elephant does, because the bones in his neck were fused, more so than those of ordinary men" (5). If this were so, and not simply a myth, it's likely that the Buddha had what is known as a "bamboo spine" (Fig. 2.3), a spine incapable of bending or turning because its numerous moveable parts, the vertebrae, have fused into a rigid, bamboo-like rod. The disorder most often responsible for such fusion is "ankylosing spondylitis," a chronic inflammatory disorder of unknown cause. Although the spine is its principal target, the aorta and the aortic valve sometimes are also attacked (17). Therefore, if the Buddha did have ankylosing spondylitis, as suggested by his having to turn his whole body around to look backwards and also by the backache(s) for which Jivaka treated him, he would have been predisposed to heart failure resulting from a deformed aortic valve. His extra teeth, the lump on his forehead, and

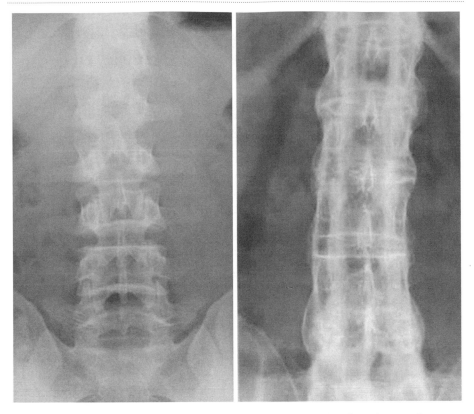

FIGURE 2.3 X-ray appearance of a "bamboo" spine (right) compared to that of a normal spine (left).

his webbed digits, while odd, were not indicative of any serious underlying disorder.

Cunda's meal must be considered a prime suspect in the investigation into the cause of death of the Buddha, given its close temporal relationship with the death. The Buddha is said to have eaten a quantity of *sūkara-maddava* almost immediately preceding the onset of his fatal attack. Unfortunately, the proper translation of the term is debated. After careful study, R. Gordon Wasson (3) concluded that *sūkara-maddava* was actually *pūtika* (*Scleroderma hydrometrica*), a species of mushroom that flourishes during northern India's rainy season and is considered a delicacy by the *Sūdra*, the lowly caste to which Cunda belonged. *Pūtika* stinks if not eaten or buried in a hole soon after harvested. According to Wasson, this is why the Buddha instructed Cunda to bury whatever was left over. Wasson also maintains that the Buddha claimed that only he could "properly assimilate" the *sūkara-maddava*, because unlike his disciples, he no longer adhered to the strict prohibition against eating mushrooms observed by Hindus of the upper castes. Since *S. hydrometrica* is not toxic, Wasson believes that the Buddha was not poisoned but died of "natural causes." The argument against mushroom poisoning as the cause of the Buddha's death is supported further by the fact that victims of such poisoning are seized by sudden appalling abdominal pain, vomiting, and sometimes bloody diarrhea, but generally no sooner than 6 to 24 hours after ingestion. This is because of the time required for the poisonous mushroom to be digested and absorbed, and its toxin to reach its site of action (18).

According to the Pali Canon, the Buddha's fatal attack involved both excruciating pain (of unspecified location) and *lohita-pakkhandika* (dysentery or "bloody flux") (13). That being the case, an infection of the large intestine (i.e., bacillary dysentery) by an invasive bacterium such as *Shigella dysenteriae*, *Salmonella enteritidis*, or entero-invasive *Escherichia coli* must be considered. Such infections are typically food-borne, increase in frequency during the rainy season in Third World countries when privies are prone to overflow, and can be severe, even rapidly fatal. However, because of the time required for such bacteria to invade the intestine (the incubation period), they do not produce symptoms until 6 to 48 hours after ingestion. Moreover, fever is typically a dominant feature of such infections, which the Buddha apparently did not have (19).

Of all the possible causes of the Buddha's fatal illness, none fits his case history better than advanced atherosclerosis of the arteries of his heart and/or his intestines. As Thomas Sydenham, "the English Hippocrates," observed over 300 years ago: "A man is as old as his arteries." The Buddha's arteries were certainly old, having suffered the wear and tear of 80 years of ascetic living, as well as the adverse effects of 6 years of starvation and likely also additional damage inflicted by a chronic inflammatory disorder (ankylosing spondylitis). The attacks of excruciating pain of unspecified location might well have been episodes of recurrent angina pectoris (cardiac pain due to poor circulation) culminating in a massive, fatal myocardial infarction. However, neither angina pectoris nor heart attacks are associated with bloody diarrhea. Therefore, if the Pali scripture is factual, and it is difficult to comprehend why the Buddha's utterly devoted followers would have invented his medical history, the *Tathāgata*'s attacks of pain were more likely abdominal angina than angina pectoris. His fatal event was more likely an infarction of the bowel than one of the heart.

Abdominal angina, recurrent abdominal pain resulting from impaired blood flow to a segment of intestine, generally is a consequence of extensive atherosclerosis of the abdominal arteries. Such pain typically begins 15 to 30 minutes after meals and lasts no more than a few hours. During this period, blood flow to the intestine normally increases in response to a heightened demand for oxygen and nutrients to support the work of digestion. In patients with abdominal angina, extensive atherosclerosis of intestinal arteries prevents this necessary increase in blood flow. Pain develops because insufficient oxygen is delivered to the intestines during this period of heightened activity. Patients quickly discover the relationship between meals and their pain and develop a fear of eating. They begin to refuse food and lose weight. Most are elderly and have generalized atherosclerosis. Their abdominal pain may persist for weeks to months before they seek medical attention or experience an intestinal catastrophe. The catastrophe, when it arrives, is manifested by the abrupt onset of intense lower abdominal pain and bloody diarrhea, often immediately following a meal. Vomiting and fever can also develop but are less common. The cause of the catastrophe is an infarction of a segment of the intestine (most often the colon) that has died because of inadequate blood flow. If the ischemia is not relieved in time or the dead segment of bowel not resected, it dissolves into a bloody pulp. Death ensues either because of a massive intestinal hemorrhage or sepsis caused by bacteria entering the bloodstream through the infarcted colonic wall (20).

The Buddha's case history is nearly classic for abdominal angina that progressed over 3 months to an infarction of the intestine. He had at least two attacks of what appear to have been abdominal angina, and one wonders if there were others preceding the final fatal one. Although the location of his pain is not recorded in the Pali text, given the bloody diarrhea that accompanied the terminal event, it was almost certainly abdominal in location. The temporal relationship between the meal served by Cunda and the fatal attack suggests, though certainly does not prove, that the meal precipitated the attack, and that other attacks of lesser severity were also likely associated with meals. Finally, the Buddha's delirium and "exceedingly bright" (white and shiny) skin just before he died are consistent with an intestinal hemorrhage so massive that it left him both confused and deathly pale.

For 80 years, the Buddha endeavored to show his followers the way to salvation by personal example. He espoused the value of a virtuous life and lived as he preached. However, "nature abhors the old" (21), and when the years had turned the Buddha into a worn-out cart, neither his extraordinary willpower nor his steadfast devotion to the virtuous life could postpone his appointment with *mahāparinirvāna*.

References

1. Carus P. *The History of the Devil and the Idea of Evil*. Whitefish, MT: Kessinger Publishing, 1900:104.

2. Keown D. *Buddhism. A Very Short Introduction*. Oxford: Oxford University Press, 1996:16–30.

3. Wasson RG. The last meal of the Buddha. *J Am Oriental Soc* 1982;102(4):591–603.

4. *Lalitavistara Sūtra. The Voice of the Buddha. The Beauty of Compassion*. Vol. I. Berkeley: Dharma Publishing, 1983:155–157, 234–235.

5. *Buddhist-Sūtras* (Davids TWR, translator). Oxford: Clarendon Press, 1881:64.

6. Op. cit. Lalitavistara Sūtra, pp. 386–390.

7. Chen TSN, Chen PSY. Jivaka, physician to the Buddha. *J Med Biography* 2002;10:88–91.

8. Op. cit. Buddhist-Sūtras, pp. 34, 35, 37.

9. Ibid., pp. 70–72.

10. Ibid., pp. 72–78.

11. Ibid., pp. 81.

12. Ibid., pp. 83.

13. Ibid., pp. 114–116.

14. Peel M. Hunger strikes. *BMJ* 1997;315:829–830.

15. Lieberson AD. How long can a person survive without food? *Scientific American*, November 8, 2004 (www.scientificamerican.com/article.cfm?id=how-long-can-a-person-sur)

16. Sparen P, Vagero D, Shestov DB, et al. Long-term mortality after severe starvation during the siege of Leningrad: prospective cohort study. *BMJ* 2004;328:11–14.

17. Taurog JD. The spondyloarthritides. In Longo DL, Fauci AS, Kasper DL, et al., eds. *Harrison's Principals of Internal Medicine*, 18th ed. New York: McGraw-Hill Medical, 2012:2774–2785.

18. Mackowiak PA. *Post Mortem. Solving History's Great Medical Mysteries*. Philadelphia: ACP Press, 2007:119.

19. Lima AAM, Guerrant RL. Inflammatory enteritides. In Mandell GL, Bennett JE, Dolin R, eds. *Principles and Practice of Infectious Diseases*, 7th ed. Philadelphia: Churchill Livingstone Elsevier, 2010:1389–1398.

20. Jacobson ED, Stephens JK, Levine JS. Mesenteric ischemia. In Yamad T, Alpers DH, Laine L, et al., eds. *Textbook of Gastroenterology*, 3rd ed. Philadelphia: Lippincott Williams & Wilkins, 1999:2583–2604.

21. Emerson RW. Circles. In: *Essays: First Series*.

3 Little Boots

OF ALL THE emperors of ancient Rome, none surpassed this patient's reputation for brutality, sadism, and perversion. He was a Julio-Claudian, a descendent of two of the most powerful families of ancient Rome —the Julians and the Claudians. Julius Caesar was his great-great-great-great uncle, Augustus his great-grandfather, and Tiberius his grandfather. His family produced six emperors who presided over Rome during perhaps its most intense period of imperial expansion, domination, and exploitation. Although brief, and in many ways overshadowed by those of his relatives, this patient's reign was not historically insignificant. During it, he formulated plans for the conquest of Britain, which came to fruition 2 years after his death during the reign of his uncle Claudius. He also instigated the first serious outbreak of anti-Semitism in the Roman world. However, his most profound impact on Roman history came from the manner of his accession. Almost immediately after the death of Tiberius, a compliant senate made him the first Roman emperor in the full sense of the title, one with unlimited powers over most of the civilized world. The senate soon came to regret so precipitously handing over supreme power to this personable but totally inexperienced young man. However, the precedent was set, and for the next four centuries his pattern of accession would be repeated again and again (1).

The patient was born on August 31, 12 CE, in Antium (Anzio), or possibly Ambitarvium (a German village just above the junction of the Rhine and Moselle rivers) (2, 3). His father, Germanicus Julius Caesar (Germanicus), was a successful and immensely popular military commander who defeated the king of Armenia and reduced Cappadocia to provincial status (4). The patient was with him on the

Rhine frontier from the age of 2 to 4 years and appears to have been something of a pampered mascot, parading around military camps dressed in miniature army attire. Germanicus' troops nicknamed him "little boots," after the tiny military boots he wore (2, 5).

His mother, Agrippina the Elder, a granddaughter of Augustus, was fiercely protective of the six of her nine children who survived infancy (6). This was an admirable trait; however, it was also one that eventually contributed to her death and those of her two oldest sons (7).

The patient had delicate health as a child. He was prone to fainting, possibly seizures, which were concerning enough to Augustus that he appointed two doctors to accompany the youngster when he traveled north to join his parents. The fainting spells troubled the patient throughout his early childhood and are reported to have made it difficult for him to stand and to walk (8). He apparently outgrew them but remained high-strung and nervous as an adult, when insomnia and headaches were responsible for some of his most intense suffering. Suetonius, one of several biographers, claims that he never managed to sleep more than 3 hours on any given night and would wander through his apartments calling for the dawn. When he did sleep, he was plagued by vivid nightmares. It was also said that during thunderstorms he became so frightened he would hide under his bed, though some modern historians doubt the veracity of this report (8, 9).

As an adult, the patient was pale and prematurely bald, although (idealized) images produced during his reign show him with a rich head of hair. His eyes were hollow, and his forehead was broad. He was uncommonly tall with very large feet, which contributed to a general lack of coordination (8, 10).

In 18–19 CE, when the patient was just 6 years old, he accompanied his father to the East. Shortly after arriving in Antioch, Germanicus suspected he was being poisoned. He died a short time later. According to Suetonius, dark stains covered his body and foam was exuding from his mouth. When his heart was found intact among his bones following cremation, murder seemed certain, given the belief that a heart steeped in poison was resistant to fire (4). The Roman populace was devastated. So great was their love for the fallen warrior that the day he died they stoned temples, upset altars, threw their household gods into the street, and refused to acknowledge their newly born children (6). In Germanicus, they had seen a successor to Tiberius whom they hoped would rescue the empire from the stagnant pool into which they believed it had descended. Popular suspicion implicated Tiberius in Germanicus' death. Agrippina, harboring similar thoughts, made no secret of her hatred of the emperor. She aroused Tiberius' enmity further by obsessively promoting the interests of her children (11) to a public devoted to her as *decus patriae, solum Augusti sanguine, unicum antiquitalis specimen* ("the glory of her country, the last of Augustus' line, an unmatched example of ancient virtues") (12). Sensing conspiracy, Tiberius retaliated through Sejanus, his commander of the Praetorian Guard, with a program of unrelenting harassment that culminated in Agrippina's death (by starvation), as well as the deaths of two of her sons, one by apparent suicide and the other by starvation. The death of the patient's brother, Drusus, was especially gruesome. Just as rumors began to circulate that he was to be reconciled with Tiberius, Drusus was starved to death in his dungeon prison. During the final days of the drawn-out process, his agony was so intense he resorted to eating the stuffing of his mattress (13).

The patient was 18 when his first brother died, 21 when his mother and other brother died. When they were imprisoned, his formidable great-grandmother, Livia, the wife and suspected poisoner of Augustus, took him under her wing and introduced him to the art of guile and cunning. He called her "a Ulysses in petticoats" after the legendary arch-trickster (2). When she died, he delivered her funeral oration, though he had not yet come of age. He then lived with his paternal grandmother, Antonia, the daughter of Mark Antony, until age 18, when his family's tormenter summoned him to the island of Capri (14). Tiberius, it seems, wanted to groom the patient as his successor, a prospect enormously popular with Rome's citizenry, in no small part because of their fond memory of the young prince's father. Whatever Tiberius' antipathy toward Agrippina and her two older sons, he appeared to bear no such grudge against the patient. Indeed, a curious bond seemed to exist between the two, possibly based on shared scholarly interests. Under Tiberius' tutelage, the patient studied Latin and Greek and became something of an expert in both sacred and secular law. He developed a reputation as one of the finest orators of his day, wrote a book on oratory, and composed poetry in Latin as well as Greek (15).

Curiously, the patient seemed to show no interest in the murder of his family or any hint of bitterness toward Tiberius. He uttered not a word of protest against the sentencing of his mother or the murder of his two brothers. Whatever Tiberius commanded, he performed willingly without question or complaint. He was, in fact, so timid and obsequious that Passienas, a later orator, was moved to say of him: "There was never a better slave or a worse master" (2, 14).

Tiberius' health began to fail in early March of 37 CE. Although initially he affected a robust appearance, his condition deteriorated rapidly with chills and pain in his side. When his end came on March 16, rumors of foul play began to circulate almost immediately. Tacitus (see below) claims that shortly after Tiberius appeared to have died, the patient, surrounded by a congratulatory crowd, stepped forth to begin his reign. But then, suddenly, Tiberius seemed to recover and was asking for food to strengthen him after a fainting spell. In the panic that ensued,

Macro, Sejanus' replacement as commander of the Praetorian Guard, calmly ordered the old man smothered with a heap of bedclothes (16, 17). In this manner, the old regime gave way to the new.

Thanks to quick work by Macro, who, like Sejanus, later would be executed for conspiring against his emperor, the patient was recognized almost immediately as Tiberius' successor. This time, in contrast to Tiberius' accession, there was a minimum of dissension among legions posted on the frontier. The magic of Germanicus' name, combined with Macro's brilliantly managed accession, created nearly universal enthusiasm for the young prince (16). As a result, in a single day, the senate granted the patient all of the honors Augustus had with difficulty been induced to accept one at a time during the long extent of his reign (18). Virtually overnight, this inexperienced and largely unknown youngster, brought up under a series of aged and repressive guardians, became master of the known world, primarily on the basis of his father's popularity (19).

In spite of his inexperience, the patient seems to have ruled admirably during the early months of his reign (18). One of his first acts was to sail through rough weather for Pandateria and the Pontian islands to fetch the ashes of his mother and brother, Nero, for proper burial in Rome (18, 20). He then turned his attention to ruling the empire. Under his influence, the aggressive Parthian King Artaganus was dissuaded from invading Syria. The patient abolished the charge of *maiestas*, a vague category of crimes concerned with general incompetence, which had been a major source of fear and resentment under Tiberius. In an enlightened act of reconciliation, he proclaimed that he harbored no animosity toward those involved in the attacks on his family and in the forum publically burned all of the papers and letters related to their cases (21, 22). So that posterity would not be deprived of important historical information, he rehabilitated the works of Titus Labienus, Cremutius Cordus, and Cassius Severus, three prominent writers long suppressed by senatorial decree (21, 23). He created a fifth judicial division to aid jurors in keeping abreast of their work; honored faithfully and uncritically every one of the bequests in Tiberius' will, though they had been ignored by the senate (24); abolished the half-percent auction tax; and compensated many families whose houses had been destroyed by fire (25).

All of these actions created a general sense of euphoria during the first months of his reign. Initially, he seemed as wise and considerate in small things as in large matters. During races, he did not signal the charioteers himself, as was his privilege, but simply viewed the spectacle seated among family and friends. He allowed those who wished to come to games barefoot to do so; senators were permitted to sit on cushions instead of bare boards; and he dispensed with formal recognition while traveling in public (26). However, the young emperor paid a heavy price for his enlightened early rule. The duties of the office and the constant public attention placed an enormous strain on his nerves and stamina, all the more so because of his former life far from public view. Hardly was his first summer in office over when he fell seriously ill 8 months after his accession (27).

The patient's illness was serious, lasting nearly a month. Many feared it would kill him. Anxious crowds besieged the palace, some swearing to fight as gladiators if only the gods would spare the young emperor's life. Others carried placards volunteering to die in his stead if necessary, so great was their love for him (21). Although there has been much speculation as to the cause of his illness, none of the historical records describe its signs or symptoms. Whatever its etiology, the patient emerged from the illness a changed man. Whereas before the illness he had been temperate and reasonable, in its aftermath he became wildly intemperate in food and drink and pleasures of the flesh (27). Because his behavior changed so radically following the illness, some historians have proposed, *post hoc ergo propter hoc*, that the illness was responsible for the change in behavior (28).

It has been said that "those whom God wishes to destroy, he first makes mad" (*Quos deus vult perdere prius dementes*). Such would appear to have been the case with this patient. Following his illness (? nervous breakdown), he was different—some might say mad. He seemed to lack any sense of proportion; exhibited delusional behavior and irrational acts; was prone to fits of megalomania and unbridled brutality; perhaps worst of all from his countrymen's perspective, he was reported to have had incestuous relations with each of his three sister (18, 29), all of which eventually led to his destruction. But was he mad?

The patient had four wives and was accused of having had homosexual relations with Marcus Aemilius Lepidus, the husband of his favorite sister, Drusilla, as well as with the comedian Mnester and various foreign hostages. He is also said to have made advances to almost every woman of rank in Rome during his brief reign (30, 31).

The patient's first wife, Junia Claudilla, died in childbirth. He married again and then again but soon tired of his next two wives and divorced them (32). His fourth and final wife, Milonia Caesonia, was neither young nor beautiful. She is said to have been recklessly extravagant and utterly promiscuous. Nevertheless, he loved her with a passionate faithfulness. He took her riding with him in helmet and cape when reviewing the troops and supposedly paraded her naked in front of friends (29). They had a daughter, on whom they both doted. They named her Julia Drusilla, after the patient's favorite sister (33). As for the rumors of incest mentioned above, even Suetonius (see below), who was prepared to believe the patient capable of almost any evil, admitted that such stories were hearsay (34).

The patient had a passion for the stage. He loved actors and enjoyed acting himself. He was a nonconformist who took great pleasure in shocking his subjects.

He enjoyed cross-dressing and wearing outrageous clothes embroidered with precious stones (35) and would appear in public carrying a thunderbolt or trident or a serpent-twined staff. He seemed to derive particular pleasure in baiting the senate, forcing some of its highest officials to run for miles beside his chariot dressed in long togas or to wait motionless in short togas at the foot of his dining couch (29). Late one night, he sent an urgent summons to the leading senators as if for some important deliberation, and when they arrived, simply danced for them (22).

On some occasions, the patient's desire to shock took the form of dark humor rooted in a theme of destructive power. During gladiatorial shows, sometimes he would have the usual equipment taken away and pit feeble old fighters against decrepit wild animals or stage comic duels between respectable householders who happened to be physically disabled in one way or other (36). Another example of his morbid sense of humor involved his explaining to a group of consuls that he had burst into sudden peals of laughter in their presence over the thought that with a single nod, he could have their throats cut (37).

The patient's lack of proportion was most striking in the attention he gave to his horse, Incitatus. He kept it in a marble stable with a stall of ivory and clothed it in purple coverlets and a collar studded with precious stones. The horse dined with him and was served its feed in fine vessels. He intended to make Incitatus a consul but didn't live long enough to follow through with his plan (35, 38, 39).

The patient insisted on being treated as a god (22, 40, 41). He impersonated Hercules, Bacchus, and all of the other divinities, not merely male but also female, often taking the role of Juno, Diana, or Venus (40). He had the heads of the most prominent statues of Greek deities, including those of Zeus and Olympia, replaced with his own bust (42). In the third year of his reign, he decided to dedicate the temple of Jerusalem to himself in the guise of Jupiter (43). Although the *genius* of living emperors had been worshipped regularly throughout the empire, especially in the eastern provinces, this would have been the first time worship of an emperor was required of the Jews. Moreover, in gross departure from tradition, he promoted a similar practice in Rome itself, where he had a temple built in which a life-sized golden image of himself was dressed each day in the same clothes he happened to wear (42, 44). Caesonia and his uncle, Claudius, were inducted into its priesthood, as was the patient himself, along with Incitatus. When the moon was full, the patient reportedly invited the Moon Goddess to his bed for sexual intercourse (42, 45). In addition, he is said to have had whispered conversations with Jupiter during the day, in which he pressed his ear to the god's mouth and sometimes raised his voice in anger (42). Some believe these were clear manifestations of an evolving insanity, others nothing more than his immature desire to behave outrageously (46).

In 40 CE, the patient mounted a military campaign against Britain, which he decided to command personally. With troops in battle formation on the Gallic side of the Channel and siege engines at ready, he put to sea in a trireme only to sail back again, seat himself on a high platform, and then give the order for his troops to begin gathering seashells in their helmets and tunics. This "plunder" he had sent to Rome as evidence of a great victory (47–49).

To these seemingly irrational acts were added ones indicative of a deep-seated megalomania, the most notorious example of which involved the construction of a bridge of boats 3.5 miles long across the Bay of Naples from Puteoli to the vicinity of Baiae. To accomplish the feat, he collected all available merchant ships and anchored them in two lines, side by side, and had earth heaped on their planks to create a kind of maritime Appian Way. The day the bridge was completed he donned the breastplate of Alexander and an oak crown and crossed to Puteoli. The next day he appeared in a charioteer's outfit driving a team of victorious race horses and followed by the entire Praetorian Guard. When the sea remained smooth and tranquil both while the bridge was being constructed and throughout the events that followed, he declared that it was because Neptune feared him (50). Some sources claim that the patient built his bridge to surpass Xerxes' feat of bridging the narrower Hellespont, others that he did so as a warning to the Germans and the Britons, on whom he had his eye. Others contend that he built it to repudiate Thrasyllus' prediction that "he had no more chance of becoming Emperor than of riding a horse dry-shod across the Gulf of Baiae" (25).

Philo of Alexandria, a Jewish historian and contemporary, was convinced that the patient was insane. He met with the patient in 40 CE as a member of a Jewish delegation that had traveled to Rome to seek the emperor's assistance in resolving a bitter dispute between Jews and Greeks living in Egypt. The hearings took place in the imperial palace, which was then under construction. During the hearing, the patient rushed from room to room, forcing the petitioners to follow while he gave instructions to his decorators (51). When he addressed the delegation, it was to ridicule them for their laws and customs (52) and to rebuke them for failing to recognize his divinity (53). When they tried to turn the discussion to their grievances, he seemed more concerned with his artwork than their political rights (51).

All of this, however, was simply theater of the absurd compared to stories of the patient's sadistic cruelty. According to some authorities, he poisoned his own grandmother, Antonia, who had taken him in when Tiberius imprisoned his mother. Moreover, when she was dead, he showed so little respect that he watched her funeral pyre burn while seated in his dining room (18, 42). He is also supposed to have forced his father-in-law to cut his own throat for not following his ship when it put to sea in a storm (42) and to have had a slave's hands cut off and hung around his neck with a placard describing his crime of having stolen a strip of silver plating from a couch (36). Many men of decent families are said to have been branded by the patient's command and sent down to the galleys or thrown to wild beasts. Others were confined in narrow cages, where they had to crouch on all fours like wild animals, or were sawn in half—and not necessarily for major offenses, but merely for criticizing his shows or failing to swear by his *genius* (36). When a knight (*eques*), on the verge of being thrown to wild beasts, shouted that he was innocent, allegedly the patient had the knight's tongue cut out and then ordered the sentence to be completed (36). On another occasion, a gladiator against whom he was fencing with a wooden sword fell down deliberately, whereupon the patient drew a real dagger and stabbed him to death. He then ran about waving the palm branch of victory (36). It is said that he advocated killing a person slowly so that he would know he was dying (36); spoke of eliminating whole legions, the senate in its entirety, and the legal profession (54); opened a brothel in his Palatine residence staffed by the children and wives of noble families to raise cash to support his extravagant lifestyle (55); sent people poisoned cakes for having reneged on bequests (56); wished that the Roman populace had a single neck so that he could break it with one swipe (36, 57); threatened to torture his wife, Caesonia; and commented when kissing his mistress' neck that he could have it slit with a single order (37). Once when there was a shortage of condemned criminals to be given to wild beasts, he is even said to have ordered some spectators thrown to them after having their tongues cut out to silence their screams (58). And after he was murdered, two books were supposedly found among his papers, each containing the names and addresses of men he had planned to kill. A huge chest of his bursting with poisons was also discovered. When Claudius later had the chest cast into the sea, enormous numbers of dead fish reportedly washed onto neighboring beaches (8). If even half of these stories were true, it's no wonder the patient died an unnatural death.

He was 24 and had ruled for a mere 3 years, 10 months, and 8 days when his end came (59). Neither the full complement of his assassins nor their precise motives are known for certain. On the fateful day, a statue of Jupiter at Olympia, which the patient had ordered moved to Rome, is said to have burst out in laughter, causing the workmen trying to dismantle it to flee. That same morning the patient, in high spirits, entered the crowded temporary theater on the Palatine. He was splashed with blood when he sacrificed a flamingo in honor of Augustus just before taking his seat. Although his habit was to leave the show at midday to bathe and have lunch, this day he lingered, possibly because of stomach troubles caused by excesses the previous night. His assassins, fearing their opportunity might slip away, contemplated attacking him where he sat. Finally, however, the emperor was persuaded to leave. The crowd was restrained to prevent them from intervening at the critical moment.

For some unknown reason the patient decided on a shorter route to the baths than that taken by his retinue. As he left the theater, he entered a narrow unguarded passageway, where he met a group of young performers from the province of Asia, who were rehearsing. He engaged them in conversation and asked them to perform for him. It was at this moment that Cassius Chaerea, tribune of the Praetorian Guard, asked him for the watchword, drew his sword, and then slashed the patient between the neck and shoulder. The emperor groaned in agony and tried to escape as his litter-bearers courageously tried to fend off several assailants with their litter poles. In the ensuing mêlée, the patient was stabbed no fewer than 30 times in a practical demonstration of the fallacy of his belief in his own divinity (59–61). *Sic semper tyrannis.* Caius Iulius Gaius Caesar (Gaius) (Fig. 3.1)—Caligula ("little boots")—was dead.

Later, the assassins went for Caesonia. They found her lying by her husband's corpse, stained with his blood, their daughter, Drusilla, by her side. They stabbed her to death and then murdered her tiny daughter by bashing her head against a wall (59, 62).

Caligula has been given various diagnoses to explain his apparent deviant behavior. His ancient biographers, Seneca, Philo, Suetonius, and Dio, all seem to have believed he was insane. However, they were historians, not physicians, and provided no precise descriptions of their subject's signs or symptoms, nor did they have the experience or the training to diagnose him.

Seneca the Younger (1–65 CE) was witness to the events of Caligula's reign and likely knew the emperor personally. However, he made a career of obsequious flattery of living emperors and unfettered vilification of dead predecessors such as Caligula. Philo (~30 BCE–45 CE), another contemporary of Caligula, as noted above, was a native of Alexandria preoccupied with problems affecting the Judean community in Alexandria. In his writings, he makes no attempt to conceal his hostility toward Caligula, whom he blamed for his people's trouble with the Greeks of Egypt. Gaius Suetonius Tranquillus (70–130 CE) and Cassius Dio (164–229 CE), two of the most important sources of the reign of Caligula, both had a tendency to believe, or at least to record, the worst about the emperor, embellishing their accounts liberally with colorful anecdotes that reflected badly on him. Neither made any serious effort to distinguish what was plausible from what was absurd. As a consequence, the accounts of each of Caligula's biographers reek of rumor, invective, and outright lies. Dio even confessed that in the telling of the emperor's story, many things that did not happen are reported, many that did happen are not reported, and everything is reported differently from how it happened. For these reasons, any attempt

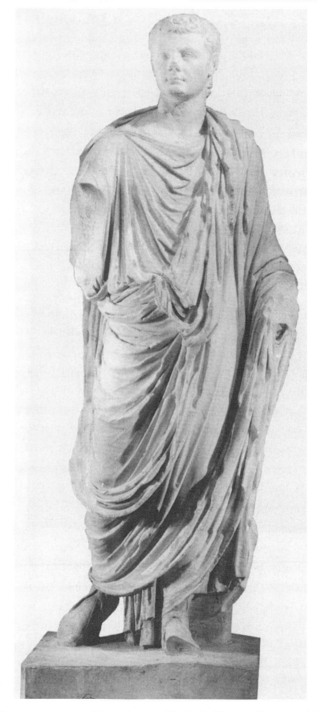

FIGURE 3.1 First-century CE marble sculpture of Caligula (Virginia Museum of Fine Arts).

to characterize, analyze, much less diagnose Caligula's psychiatric disorder, if in fact he had one, is largely an exercise in separating fact from falsehood (63).

The fundamental question first posed by the ancients is: Was Caligula mad? Certainly, there is considerable evidence of abnormal behavior, at least by modern standards, in his historical record. If the various anecdotes related above have any basis in fact, he exhibited socially outrageous behavior, delusions of grandeur, bizarre and irrational acts, sleep disturbance, paraphilias (i.e., sexual deviation), and recurrent headaches. Such behavior was regarded as abnormal during his lifetime, probably no less so than today, but in what way? How did the Romans conceptualize aberrant behavior, and how did such concepts differ from those of today?

Our information on the practice of medicine in 1st-century CE Rome comes largely from Celsus, a contemporary of Caligula. He was not a physician but an intelligent layman with an interest in medicine. His work *De Medicina* (On Medicine) is the principal surviving part of an encyclopedia he wrote on agriculture, military art, rhetoric, philosophy, and jurisprudence (64). In *De Medicina*, he described several classes of mental illness, along with their treatments. These included acute insanity (*insania*), epilepsy (*morbus comitialis*), and lethargy (65). "Vain imaginings" in the absence of frank delirium characterized acute insanity, of which there were sad (*tristis*) and hilarious (*hilaris*) forms. Celsus also called attention to a distinction between febrile and nonfebrile varieties of insanity and the fact that the former was associated with a poorer prognosis (66). Prolonged insanity, which was believed to result from an excess of black bile (*melancholia*), was likely the disorder we call "chronic depression" today (67). This type of insanity had depressed as well as hilarious subtypes, possibly indicative of the present-day diagnosis of manic depression. According to Celsus, the latter, which was frequently associated with excess laughter, had the better prognosis (68).

Treatment of these disorders, then as now, was multimodal as well as multidisciplinary. Patients suffering from *insania* were thought to respond better to a light than a dark environment. Application of warm liquids (*fomentum*) to the body and shaving the head were recommended, as were treatments with various roots, draughts, and purgatives. Clysters (enemas) were popular as treatments for both physical and mental disorders. Some treatments were phase- and symptom-specific, as for example the use of music to treat *melancholia*. When patients exhibited *vanae imagines*, caregivers were urged to agree with, rather than oppose, them. However, if these were disabling, certain "tortures" (*tormenta*) were recommended. Such treatments, which included starvation, fettering, flogging, and forced memorization, were not likely to have been any better received by patients of Caligula's day than treatments such as electroconvulsive therapy (ECT) are today (69).

To the extent that the description of Caligula's disordered behavior by the ancient historians is valid, a physician subscribing to the medical doctrine described by Celsus likely would have diagnosed the emperor with acute, nonfebrile insanity of the hilarious type; a good prognosis would have been predicted. The same doctor might have entertained, as an alternative diagnosis, insanity caused by a love potion or "philter" (see below). Since Caligula's insanity appeared to incline him to violence, torture would have been considered an appropriate treatment, as would have been the administration of a clyster (69). How inclined a physician might have been to attempt such treatments on a monarch of Caligula's disposition is a matter for the reader's speculation.

Thanks to recent advances in the science of the brain, we now believe that the causes of most psychiatric disorders derive from deviant patterns of brain development and/or defective neurotransmitters, deranged gene expression, or adverse hormonal influences on brain function. These concepts evolved as a result of spectacular discoveries by neuroscientists beginning in the late 20th century, which made it possible to explain brain–behavior relationships in terms of neuroanatomy and neurochemistry. Unfortunately, even today, the essential question regarding the cause of deviant behaviors remains unanswered, and modern concepts, in this regard, are no less speculative than those of the ancients.

This is not to say that modern clinicians are incapable of diagnosing (i.e., giving a name to) Caligula's disorder; for today, as in ancient Rome, psychiatric diagnoses are mainly descriptive in spite of the modern advances in brain science. Today, such diagnoses are based on criteria enumerated in the fourth edition of a manual developed by the American Psychiatric Association called the *Diagnostic and Statistical Manual of Mental Disorders IV* (DSM-IV) (70).

Even at his worst, as depicted by the ancient historians, Caligula does not meet the DSM-IV criteria for a major psychosis. There is no evidence that he had auditory hallucinations, exhibited disorganized or catatonic behavior, or had a flat or inappropriate affect. Therefore, although at times he seems to have exhibited paranoia, he was not a paranoid schizophrenic.

If Caligula did have a psychiatric disorder, most likely it was one of two personality disorders—the antisocial personality disorder or the narcissistic personality disorder (Table 3.1). With regard to the former, as characterized by the ancient historians, he was clearly impulsive, irritable, aggressive, and remorseless. He exhibited a flagrant disregard for social norms and had a reckless disregard for the safety of others. However, he did not exhibit such deviant behavior until he became emperor at 20 years of age.

With regard to the narcissistic personality disorder, he was certainly grandiose, exploitative, unempathetic, and arrogant. He fantasized that he was a god and demanded to be worshipped as such. His sense of entitlement was extraordinary.

TABLE 3.1

Hyphen: DSM-IV Criteria Defining Antisocial and Narcissistic Personality Disorders

A. 301.7 ANTISOCIAL PERSONALITY DISORDER*

Pervasive pattern of violation of the rights of others

1. Failure to conform to social norms
2. Deceitfulness
3. Impulsivity
4. Irritability and aggressiveness
5. Reckless disregard for safety of self or others
6. Irresponsibility (e.g., regarding finances)
7. Lack of remorse (for having injured another)

*Evidence of disordered conduct before age 15 years

B. 301.81 NARCISSISTIC PERSONALITY DISORDER

Grandiosity, need for admiration, and lack of empathy

1. Grandiose, expects to be recognized as superior
2. Fantasies of unlimited success, power, brilliance, beauty
3. Believes that he/she is "special" and unique
4. Requires excessive admiration
5. Sense of entitlement, unreasonable expectations of automatic compliance
6. Interpersonally exploitative
7. Lacks empathy
8. Envious of others or believes other envious of him/her
9. Arrogant, haughty

Even so, many of these *abnormal* personality traits were exhibited by other emperors of ancient Rome.

Today, given Caligula's symptoms, he would likely receive any one of a number of antipsychotic drugs to manage his antisocial outbursts and an antidepressant for melancholic periods (if diagnosed). Lithium or one of the other antiseizure medications might be used to stabilize his mood and behavior, anti-anxiety drugs to mollify his response to stress. Hypnotic drugs would be given to help him sleep and analgesics to alleviate his headaches. Psychosocial counseling would be added to this panoply of medications in an effort to reduce stress, enhance interpersonal relations, eliminate substance abuse, and control anger.

Although diagnosing either of these personality disorders would enable the clinician to pigeonhole Caligula among other patients with similar symptoms, it would offer no insight into the cause of his disorder. To paraphrase Shakespeare (*Julius Caesar* I, ii 148), it would not reveal upon what meat this, our Caesar, fed, that he grew so antisocial/narcissistic.

Some believe it was the meat of absolute power that corrupted Caligula. They support this conclusion by pointing to examples throughout history (e.g., Nero, Ivan the Terrible, Saddam Hussein) in which absolute power of the kind wielded by Caligula is thought to have led from "free indulgence in sensual pleasures to immoderate lust and debauchery, to domination, contempt and pleasure in suffering, to final derangement" (71). Add to this phenomenon the violent times in which Caligula ruled and the constant threat of assassination under which he lived, and his "antisocial" behavior is readily explained on the basis of an appropriate response to threat.

Many of Caligula's symptoms were also characteristic of posttraumatic stress disorder (PTSD), especially his substance abuse (see below), headaches, insomnia, nightmares, and fear of thunderstorms (72). To be sure, he was subjected to an extraordinary number of severe traumatic events throughout his brief life. His father died (probably poisoned) when he was 6. Drusus, Tiberius' son, who became his surrogate father, died (also probably poisoned) when Caligula was 11 (73). Titus Sabinus, another loyal friend of the family, was executed and had his body hurled down the Gemonian Stairs and flung into the Tiber when Caligula was 16 (74). When he was 18, his brother Nero was executed under circumstances arranged to look like suicide (75). Shortly after Caligula's first marriage at age 21, his wife and unborn daughter died in childbirth (32). And 4 years before becoming emperor, he endured the gruesome deaths of his mother and other brother (13). The combined effect of these repeated major traumatic events, beginning as they did in early childhood and continuing through adolescence, would be more than sufficient to produce florid PTSD in the average person.

Of the other diagnoses given to Caligula, none fits his clinical profile as well as that of a personality disorder complicated by PTSD and accentuated by the influence of absolute power. Seizures seem to have been rife among the Julio-Claudians. Julius Caesar (Caligula's great-great-great-great-uncle), Julia (grandmother), Agrippina II (sister), and Britannicus (cousin) were all reported to have suffered with seizures (71). Caligula is said to have had fainting spells as a child, and it has been speculated that his aberrant behavior was the consequence of seizures—specifically ones originating in temporal lobe of the brain (Fig. 3.2). Although temporal lobe seizures can sometimes produce bizarre behavior, they would be a decidedly less likely cause of the behavior manifested by Caligula than the personality disorder described above. Moreover, because until recent times any fit, fainting spell, or sleeping spell was diagnosed as "epilepsy" (76–78), we have no way of knowing if Caligula's fainting spells were actually seizures.

It also has been speculated that Caligula's mysterious illness shortly after he became emperor was actually an attack of encephalitis (a viral infection of the

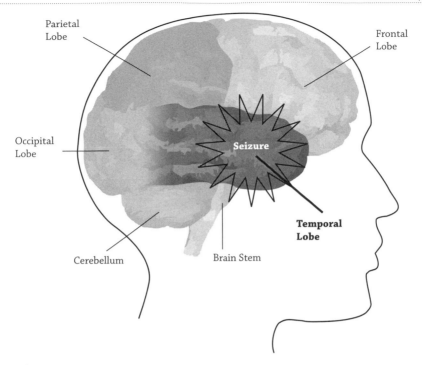

FIGURE 3.2 Drawing of the human brain showing the location of the temporal lobe in relation to the other cerebral lobes.

brain), which while not lethal, was severe enough to have disordered the function of his brain in its aftermath (71). Although instances of striking "post-encephalitic" changes in personality have been reported (79), they are exceedingly rare. Moreover, most modern historians believe the illness was actually the result of a nervous breakdown rather than an episode of encephalitis.

Both Suetonius and Philo claimed that Caligula drank a wide range of exotic beverages to excess (27, 56). There was also an ancient tradition that explained Caligula's behavior as madness caused by an aphrodisiac administered by Caesonia, his fourth, reputedly promiscuous, wife (8). However, these reports in particular must be regarded with skepticism. Caligula's biographers, as already mentioned, wrote their accounts for succeeding emperors who wished to distinguish themselves by denigrating their predecessors. Such denigration frequently took the form of moralizing rhetoric condemning predecessors for sexual misbehavior, gluttony, drunkenness, excessive spending, effeminate behavior, and the like (Joshel SR, personal communication). Unfortunately, it is not possible to know for certain when such descriptions are metaphors for political criticism or facts of behavior.

Caligula was not mad (insane) by modern standards. However, he was deeply troubled by a personality disorder complicated by a traumatized youth, a position of absolute power, and the ever-present threat of assassination (38, 80). He was not universally despised. In fact, following his assassination, the entire Germanic corps rampaged in protest, with considerable blood being shed (81). Although Seneca accused Caligula of having wasted and utterly destroyed the empire, under his stewardship the Roman provinces actually enjoyed a generally stable and orderly government; the frontiers were secure; and many prominent Romans did quite well despite a concerted effort to discredit Caligula's record afterwards. He supposedly left the empire bankrupt (8), and yet his successor, Claudius, found enough funds in the imperial treasury to be able to abolish taxes and at the same time undertake expensive building projects (1). Caligula appointed competent subordinates, especially in the East, and was generally held in awe by his subjects (82). He revived Augustus' practice, discontinued by Tiberius, of publishing an imperial budget (21) and invested magistrates with full authority to carry out their sentences without his prior approval (21). He reinitiated construction of a canal across the Isthmus of Corinth and saw to the building of a lighthouse at Boulogne to assist military transport ships traveling between the continent and Britain. He also initiated the construction of two new aqueducts to relieve Rome's inadequate supply of fresh water, as well as the Didymaean Apollo's temple at Ephesus, and completed the Temple of Augustus and Pompey's Theater, rebuilt the ancient walls and temples of Syracuse, and restored the palace at Samos (42, 82).

However, Caligula was insufferably arrogant and totally ruthless in his attacks on those he perceived to be plotting against him. One of his first acts as emperor was to put to death his cousin, Tiberius, the natural grandson of the emperor of the same name and co-claimant to the throne. When the time came for the young Tiberius to take his own life (for the law prohibited another from carrying out the execution of a descendent of an emperor), he was so naïve that the centurion in attendance had to show him where to thrust his sword (83). Caligula's provocation of the Jews marked the end of warm relations between them and Rome and the beginning of a serious and progressive deterioration of the relationship that would eventually end in the Jewish Wars and the destruction of the Temple in Jerusalem. In addition, by summoning the king of Mauretania to Rome and then executing him, Caligula instigated another senseless war with a faithful Roman ally (84).

The nature and cause of Caligula's psychopathology have long remained two of history's great unsolved mysteries, not because modern clinicians lack the expertise to give the disorder a name, but because its true character has been so difficult to glean from the conflation of rumor, invective, gossip, and fact that is the historical record. Clearly, Caligula had virtues, though likely even more vices. In death's final accounting, he was probably neither better nor worse than many of those who ruled the empire before and after him. *Requiescat in pace.*

References

1. Barrett AA. *Caligula. The Corruption of Power*. New Haven: Yale University Press, 1989:xv–xix.

2. Suetonius Tranquillas G. *Lives of the Twelve Caesars* (translated by Graves R). New York: Welcome Rain Publishers, 2001:137.

3. Taylor A. An allusion to the riddle in Suetonius. *Am J Philol* 1945;66:408–410.

4. Op. cit. Suetonius, p. 135.

5. Tacitus. *The Annals of Imperial Rome* (translated with introduction by Grant M). London: Penguin, 1996:56.

6. Op. cit. Suetonius, p. 136.

7. Op. cit. Tacitus, p. 163.

8. Op. cit. Suetonius, p. 155.

9. Op. cit. Barrett, p. 213.

10. Ibid., pp. 42–43.

11. Ibid., p. 19.

12. Ibid., p. 16.

13. Ibid., p. 31.

14. Op. cit. Tacitus, p. 209.

15. Op. cit. Barrett, p. 47.

16. Op. cit. Suetonius, pp. 137–138.

17. Op. cit. Tacitus, pp. 225–226.

18. Dio, Cassius. *Roman History, Book 59*. Available online at http://penelope.uchicago.edu/Thayer/E/Roman/Texts/Cassius_Dio/home.html, p. 3.

19. Op. cit. Barrett, pp. 54–57.

20. Op. cit. Suetonius, p. 139.

21. Ibid., p. 140.

22. Op. cit. Dio, pp. 4–5.

23. Op. cit. Barrett, pp. 63–65.

24. Op. cit. Dio, p. 2.

25. Op. cit. Suetonius, pp. 142–143.

26. Op. cit. Dio, p. 6.

27. Philo J. On the Embassy to Gaius. In *The Works of Philo Judaeus. The Contemporary of Josephus* (translated from Greek by Yonge CD). Available online at http://www.earlychristianwritings.com/yonge/index-2.html, p. 2.

28. Op. cit. Barrett, p. 73.

29. Op. cit. Suetonius, p. 144.

30. Ibid., p. 150.

31. Op. cit. Dio, p. 9.

32. Op. cit. Barrett, pp. 34, 77, 89.

33. Ibid., pp. 94–96.

34. Ibid., p. 85.

35. Ibid., pp. 43, 46.

36. Op. cit. Suetonius, p. 145–146.

37. Op. cit. Barrett, p. 241.

38. Op. cit. Suetonius, p. 156.

39. Op. cit. Dio, p. 11.

40. Ibid., p. 21.

41. Op. cit. Philo, p. 8.

42. Op. cit. Suetonius, p. 143.

43. Op. cit. Philo, p. 20.

44. Ibid., p. 35.

45. Op. cit. Dio, p. 22.

46. Op. cit. Barrett, pp. 145–147, 214–217.

47. Ibid., p. 135.

48. Op. cit. Suetonius, p. 154.

49. Op. cit. Dio, p. 19.

50. Ibid., pp. 13–14.

51. Op. cit. Philo, p. 37.

52. Ibid., p. 19.

53. Ibid., p. 36.

54. Op. cit. Suetonius, p. 148.

55. Op. cit. Dio, p. 23.

56. Op. cit. Suetonius, p. 150–151.

57. Op. cit. Dio, p. 10.

58. Ibid., p. 8.

59. Op. cit. Suetonius, p. 158.

60. Op. cit. Dio, p. 24.

61. Op. cit. Barrett, pp. 163–165.

62. Ibid., p. 166.

63. Ibid., pp. xx–xxiii.

64. Jackson R. *Doctors and Diseases in the Roman Empire*. Norman: University of Oklahoma Press, 1988:9.

65. Celsus AC. *De Medicina* (On Medicine), vol. 1, Book III. Loeb Classical Library Edition, 1935, pp. 290–304, 334–340. Available online at http://penelope.uchicago.edu/thayer/E/RomanTexts/Celsus/3*.html.

66. Ibid., p. 290.

67. Ibid., p. 300.

68. Ibid., p. 302.

69. Ibid., pp. 295–296.

70. American Psychiatric Association. *Diagnostic and Statistical Manual of Mental Disorders,* 4th ed. (DSM-IV). Washington, DC: American Psychiatric Association, 2000.

71. Sandison AT. The madness of the emperor Caligula (Gaius Julius Caesar Germanicus). *Med Hist* 1958;2:202–209.

72. Mackowiak PA. *Post Mortem. Solving History's Great Medical Mysteries*. Philadelphia: ACP Press, 2007:294–299.

73. Op. cit. Tacitus, p. 161.

74. Ibid., p. 190.

75. Op. cit. Barrett, p. 27.

76. Katz RS. The illness of Caligula. *Classical World* 1972;65:223–225.

77. Morgan MG. Caligula's illness again. *Classical World* 1973;66:327–329.

78. Benediktson DT. Caligula's madness: madness or interictal temporal lobe epilepsy? *Classical World* 1989;82:370–375.

79. McCauley MC. An artist's mind after injury. Encephalitis destroyed Lonnie Sue Johnson's memory, but whimsy and art remain. *The Baltimore Sun*. September 18, 2011, A&E section, pp. 1, 6.

80. Op. cit. Dio, p. 20.

81. Ibid., p. 25.

82. Op. cit. Barrett, p. 223.

83. Op. cit. Philo, p. 4.

84. Valente WA, Talbert RJA, Hallett JP, Mackowiak PA. Caveat cenans! *Am J Med* 2002; 112:392–398.

4 Noble Enemy

IN THE 12TH CENTURY CE, Palestine was a lightning rod for storms of conquest and counter-conquest. It was the promised land of Christian zealots seeking the kingdom of heaven and of peasants hoping to escape the oppression of aristocratic lords. It was the destination of great armies drawn from the West by greed for Oriental treasure, dreams of adventure and world dominion, and the prospect of guaranteeing a place in paradise through personal atonement. All of these sources of energy coalesced and were discharged in a series of Holy Wars known as "the Crusades" to produce some of the cruelest and bloodiest chaos the region has yet known (1).

The Crusades raged from the end of the 11th century until late in the 13th century. There were eight in all—four major and four minor. The first began in 1096 with the departure of five armies from Europe at different times. In 1098, one led by Godfrey of Bouillon stormed the Holy City, massacred the Muslim defenders by the thousands, and established the Latin Kingdom of Jerusalem. Within 30 years, Christian knights controlled the greater part of Palestine and the coast of Syria, capitalizing on divisions within the Muslim ranks. Though the thousand tribes of Arabia greatly outnumbered the Christians, they were divided into Sunni and Shi'ite sects and answered to different emirs and viziers aligned in some cases with the Fatimid caliphate of Egypt and in others with the caliphate of Baghdad. Because of these religious and political differences, infighting among the forces of Islam was nearly continuous.

The leaders of the Latin Kingdom were lesser personages of Europe—the younger sons of minor households with little future at home, who had come to the Orient in search of position, wealth, and adventure. They relied on the ferocious cavalry charge of well-armed and heavily armored knights to rout the Saracens in pitched battle, as well as a series of impressive fortresses for protection in tactical retreats. For over 90 years after the creation of their Crusader kingdom, they lived in a state of ceaseless conflict with the Arabs of the Levant. They mounted a second (unsuccessful) Crusade against Damascus in 1144. The seed of the third was planted less than half a century later, when Guy of Lusignan arrived in Jerusalem from his native Poitou (France).

Although the scion of a minor noble house, Guy was banished from Aquitaine after murdering the Earl of Salisbury as he returned from a pilgrimage to Santiago de Compestela. Bold, ambitious, and handsome, Guy successfully wooed Sibylla, the recently widowed sister of Baldwin IV, the reigning king of Jerusalem. A wise monarch, Baldwin had the misfortune of having contracted leprosy, which disfigured, blinded, and eventually killed him. Having no son, the king named his nephew as heir. With the king's condition worsening year after year and his nephew a sickly toddler, Guy was appointed regent of the realm in 1184. When the leper king died along with his tiny nephew in 1185, Guy usurped the throne and was crowned king in mid-September 1186. The following year he proved to be less of a fighter than a lover. It was then that his defeat at the Horns of Hattin gave birth to a third Crusade (2).

Of all the warriors who fought in the Crusades, none cast a larger shadow over the era than this patient—one even larger than that of his most famous adversary, Richard I ("the Lionheart"). He was the one who annihilated King Guy's army at the Horns of Hattin in 1187 and reclaimed Jerusalem for Islam (3) after it had been ruled for nearly a century by a Christian coalition of "Franks," composed of French speakers from France, Normandy, and Flanders, Normans from Sicily and Italy, knights from Spain, and small numbers of Germans and Englishmen (4). The victory solidified his position as "Sultan" and also brought Richard and Philip II (Augustus) of France to Palestine at the head of a third Crusade. When they arrived, the patient was the one who met them, denied them Jerusalem, and forced them to abandon their quest to free the Holy Land from the Muslims (2).

Although his victory over Frankish forces at Hattin was one of the most spectacular in military history, the patient became a figure of myth and legend more for his image as the "noble enemy" than for his victories on the battlefield (5). For he, more than the Christian knights who opposed him, exemplified chivalrous ideals in his conduct both as military leader and civil servant (6). Largely unfamiliar to Westerners today, he was an uncommonly charismatic warrior, revered even by his enemies for his unflagging commitment to personal honor during one of the most brutal periods in the history of the Levant. These qualities were the fountainhead of his military genius, which enabled him finally to unite, control, and direct the disparate tribes of Islam in a protracted Holy War.

The patient was born in Tikrit in 1138 (7) to a Kurdish family originating from a highland village in Greater Armenia (8). Little is known of his youth, and what information exists is contradictory (9). It is known that when he was 18, he was appointed deputy to his uncle, Shirkuh, who was then military governor of Damascus. At the age of 26, he accompanied his uncle as Quartermaster-General of a Syrian expeditionary force that defeated a Frankish-Egyptian army commanded by King Amalric at the battle of Ashmunein. It was the second of three invasions of Egypt by Syria between 1164 and 1169. The patient skillfully directed troops in action and successfully defended Alexandria during the campaign, giving the Franks their first glimpse of the generalship of the man who would harass them for the next two and a half decades (10). When Shirkuh died suddenly in 1169, he was replaced by the patient.

The patient was 30 when he assumed command of the Syrian army and began campaigning nearly continuously for over two decades. In 1171, he conquered the Fatimid rulers of Egypt, in 1174 Damascus, in 1183 the Syrian city of Aleppo, and in 1186 Mosul in Iraq. Following his victory over the Franks at Hattin in 1187, he invested one Christian fortress after another until nearly all of Palestine returned to Muslim control. Tyre, however, could not be taken, and it was there that Richard disembarked at the head of the third Crusade. Although the new Crusaders recovered Acre and several other cities from the Muslims in the 2 years that followed, the patient denied them Jerusalem. On September 2, 1192, he concluded a truce with Richard permitting Christians to visit the Holy City without paying tribute in addition to free access to the holy places (11).

Only fragments of the patient's medical history have been preserved for posterity. They were recorded by Beha Ed-din (12), a close associate and an eyewitness to events involving the Sultan from 1188 (when he was 50) until his death in 1193 (13). Though generally regarded as a credible historian, Beha Ed-din was not a physician. Moreover, his account of the patient's medical history, while lucid, is only moderately detailed.

Beha Ed-din, a native of Mosul, was the chief agent for the Zengid emir of Mosul, Izz Ed-din, during negotiations in 1186, which were to give the patient suzerainty over the city. The Sultan was so impressed by Beha Ed-din's bearing that he offered him the directorship of a college in Cairo. Beha Ed-din refused, fearing the offer would be viewed as an inducement to influence him in the patient's favor during his negotiations on behalf of Izz Ed-din. Two years later, however, he entered the Sultan's service and, although 7 years younger than the patient, became a close confidant and first-hand witness of his activities thereafter (12).

The patient's first serious illness, according to Beha Ed-din, began in December 1185, when the Sultan was 48 (14). He was besieging Mosul at the time in a third attempt to wrest control of the walled citadel from Zengi Muslims, who were then closely allied with his Frankish enemies (15). His illness lasted more than 2 months and was so severe that when Beha Ed-din saw him in late February 1186, he expected the Sultan to die. Beha Ed-din did not record the patient's signs or symptoms, although others have speculated that fever was a prominent feature of the illness. Nor do we know if other subjects or associates of the Sultan were similarly affected, in which case malaria, typhoid fever, or one of the many other gastrointestinal infections that plagued armies before the advent of modern sanitary practice would have been a likely diagnosis. Whatever the etiology of his illness, by mid-year the patient looked like "a man risen from the dead" (16).

The patient's adversaries at the time of his illness, the "Zengids," were followers of the family of Zengi, an early ruler of Mosul credited with initiating the Islamic counter-crusade with a bloody victory over the Franks just south of Aleppo in 1130. Zengi also reclaimed the ancient and rich city of Edessa from the Christians in 1144. A brutal and intemperate Turk, he waged not a Holy War per se but one in which he fought fellow Muslims as often as Christians in the interest of personal empire. The taking of Damascus (from Muslim brothers) and control of traffic between Mesopotamia, Egypt, and the Crusader states seems to have been his ultimate ambition. His followers, although proud of their Turkish heritage and their association with the family of Zengi, did not hesitate to side with one brother against another when quarrels erupted, or even change sides to gain some advantage. In 1146, Zengi was succeeded by his son, Nur Ed-din, a devout believer and good soldier, who promoted the idea of recovering Jerusalem and purifying it of nonbelievers. The security of his position as leader of the Zengids required a war against the Latin Kingdom. However, unlike the patient, he was unable to keep a sufficiently large fighting force together for the length of time required to mount an effective campaign against the Crusaders. When he died suddenly in 1174, the patient emerged as his spiritual successor and at last united Egypt and Syria in the Holy War Nur Ed-din had envisioned but had not been able to effectuate (15).

Following the above illness, the Sultan's health seems to have waxed and waned with "recurrent bouts of fever and colic" (17). Even so, he recovered sufficiently from his near-fatal disorder to lead troops personally into battle. In July 1190, for example, he was vigorous enough to respond to a surprise attack on his right wing by springing to his horse, crying, "On for Islam!" and hurling himself with his troops against the Franks "like lions springing on their prey" (18). However, in October 1190, he was again ill with an attack of what Beha Ed-din called "bilious fever" (19). The illness was severe enough to confine him to his bed and lasted well into November.

An associate, Zein Ed-din Yusuf, Lord of Arbela, was similarly affected with "two successive fevers," suggesting that both his illness and the patient's were characterized by a periodic fever and perhaps also jaundice, in which case malaria would have been their likely diagnosis. Beha Ed-din believed that the illness developed because "the air of the plain of Acre [where they were then encamped] had been made unhealthy by the great number of dead left by either side on the field" (20). "Malaria," which is Italian for "bad air," reflects its long-appreciated association with the unhealthy air of marshy areas where malaria-infested mosquitoes abound (21).

Whatever the cause of this illness or the patient's earlier one, Palestine was then a decidedly unhealthy place. Amalric, who was king of Jerusalem from 1158 until his death, succumbed to dysentery at the age of 38 in 1180, leaving control of the Latin Kingdom to his leprous son, Baldwin IV (22). Richard the Lionheart fell ill shortly after arriving at the head of the third Crusade and then again while negotiating a truce with the patient just before departing from Palestine in September 1192 (23). Virtually nothing is known of the nature of his latter illness; however, Beha Ed-din tells us that at his request, the patient provided Richard with fruit and snow (24). King Philip of France abandoned the third Crusade at least in part because of illness (character unknown). Although the Sultan was informed that he died at Antioch before he could reach home (25), in fact Philip recovered, returned to France, and immediately took up arms against the vast Plantagenet domain of his former lover, Richard (23). With regard to Crusaders of lesser station, it has been estimated that in the 2-year siege of Acre (1189–1191) alone, the Franks "lost 100,000 men, rather more from disease than in battle"; the patient's army lost far fewer (26).

The patient seems to have weathered reasonably well both his illnesses and the rigors of campaigning for two and a half decades before being overtaken by his final illness. It struck when he was 56 and already beginning to show the physical and psychological effects of the privations and trauma of unrelenting combat. By then he complained: "I am an old man now. I have no longer any desires of pleasures of the world. I have had my fill of them and have renounced them forever" (27).

When Beha Ed-din visited him in February 1193, the Sultan had lost his appetite and complained of weakness, lassitude, and indigestion. The weather was damp and cold, and yet the patient set out on horseback without the quilted tunic he always wore in public and "seemed like a man awakening from a dream." In the evening, his lassitude increased and "a little before midnight he had an attack of bilious fever, which was internal rather than external." The next day his fever was worse. However, when "it was suppressed" (by unknown means), he seemed to improve and to take pleasure in his conversation with Beha Ed-din. Nevertheless, "from that time, the Sultan's illness grew more and more serious," with headaches of mounting intensity. Those in attendance began to despair for his life, all the more so because of "the absence of his chief physician, who knew his constitution better than anyone." After having been bled on the fourth day of his illness, the patient "grew seriously worse, and the humours of the body began to cease their flow." On the sixth day, his attendants propped him into a sitting position and gave him lukewarm water "as an emollient after the medicine he had taken." During the next 2 days, his condition deteriorated as his "mind began to wander." By the ninth day of illness, he was stuporous and "unable to take the draught that was brought to him." His subjects, sensing his end was near, were "afraid and began to carry away their goods out of the Bazaars." On the tenth day, a clyster was applied twice, which seemed to give the Sultan relief. He took a few sips of barley-water. That night he began to perspire, which his attendants regarded as a hopeful sign. By the next day, "the perspiration was so profuse that it had gone right through the mattress and the mats, and the moisture could be seen on the floor." On the twelfth night, the patient grew weaker, wavering in and out of consciousness. His attendants expected him to die. However, he lingered on until the fourteenth day of illness. On Wednesday, the 27th of Safer, in the year 589 (March 4, 1193), after the hour of morning prayer, Al-Malik al-Nasir Salah al-Din Abu 'l-Muzaffer Yusuf ibn Ayyub ibn Shadi (Saladin) (Fig. 4.1) died (28). His body was laid to rest in the garden near the summerhouse of the palace in Damascus. Three years later it was placed in a mausoleum to the north of the Great Mosque (29).

The identity of the mysterious disorder that carried off Saladin is a secret not likely ever to be revealed for certain. The clinical information provided by Beha Ed-din is insufficient to render a definitive diagnosis, and yet it contains enough details to narrow the list of possibilities to just a few—ones capable of explaining a fatal illness with an acute onset and subacute course, heralded by lassitude, weakness, and indigestion, and dominated by fever (bilious?), headache, progressive disorientation, and profuse sweating.

There were many diseases for which his profession placed Saladin at particular risk. Prior to the advent of modern public health concepts and interventions, warriors were especially prone to infections caused by intestinal pathogens that circulated in army camps because of poor sanitation, arthropod-borne infections (transmitted by mosquitoes and other biting insects) endemic to campaign sites, sexually transmitted diseases, and infections whose transmission was facilitated from person to person by the crowded conditions of military encampments. Given the prevalence, diversity, and severity of the disorders confronting the armies of Saladin and his antagonists, the inadequate sanitation, and the lack of immunizations and basic medical care, one marvels that any of the participants in the Crusades survived long enough to provide posterity with a record of their experiences.

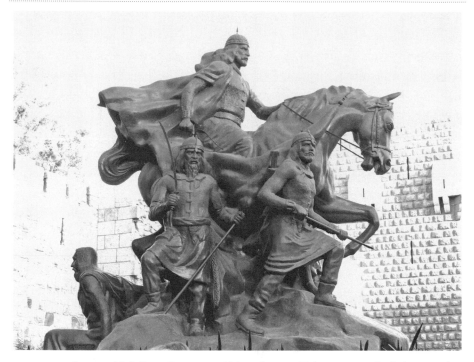

FIGURE 4.1 Statue of Saladin in Damascus. Although no real-life portraits of Saladin exist, his biographies give the impression that he was tall, dark (both by inheritance and constant exposure to the sun), bearded, and thin (having spent most of his life in the saddle and having been notoriously abstemious in his eating).

The combination of fever, headache, and progressive disorientation suggests that Saladin's fatal disorder was an infection and that its primary focus was the brain, in that headache and disorientation were the earliest manifestations of his subacute illness. Of such infections, only a few are worth considering: tuberculous meningitis (tuberculosis of the membranes surrounding the brain and spinal cord) and viral encephalitis (infections of the brain caused by herpes simplex virus, West Nile virus, or one of several other arthropod-borne viruses attacking the central nervous system).

According to Beha Ed-din, Saladin began to perspire profusely in the evening of the tenth day of his fatal illness. Physicians today would say he was having "night sweats," a phenomenon long recognized as one of the classic manifestations of advanced tuberculosis. While certainly not specific for tuberculosis, night sweats occur substantially less often during the other infections mentioned above than during tuberculosis. Moreover, tuberculosis was rampant during the medieval period (30, 31). Its high prevalence during that era is reflected in accounts of the "ceremony of the touch" performed by French and English monarchs to cure subjects suffering with scrofula, a form of tuberculosis involving the glands of the neck. The practice, which originated with Clovis in the 5th century AD, was based on the belief that at the time of their anointment, the kings of France received from God the power to heal scrofula by their touch. Edward the Confessor claimed the same healing power for English kings in the 11th century, an office that remained in England's *Book of Common Prayer* until 1719. In time, because of the practice, scrofula came to be known as the "king's evil." According to royal records, many thousands of pilgrims travelled yearly to be touched and cured by monarchs on both sides of the English Channel at the time of the Crusades. Philip Augustus, for example, is credited with 1,500 touches during a single such ceremony. Thus, Saladin lived (and died) during a time of widespread tuberculosis. Although there is no evidence that he suffered with scrofula, his terminal fever, night sweats, headaches, and progressive disorientation do suggest that he died of a different form of tuberculosis, namely tuberculous meningitis, tuberculosis of the membranes covering the brain and spinal cord.

If the "bilious fever" reported by Beha Ed-din was indicative of an illness involving both fever and jaundice, as the name implies, and also altered mentation, as evidenced later in the course of Saladin's terminal illness, an infection known as "leptospirosis" must be included among potential diagnoses. Leptospirosis is one of only a few infections that simultaneously attacks the liver and brain (32). It is a zoonosis—that is, an infection primarily of animals, which only occasionally spills over into human populations—with a worldwide distribution. It is caused by corkscrew-shaped bacteria belonging to the genus *Leptospira* (derived from the Greek *leptos* [thin] and Latin *spira* [coiled]). Although many small and large mammals are infected by *Leptospira*, rodents are the most important source of human infections, which develop as a result of contact of the urine or tissues of infected animals with cuts and abrasions or mucous membranes lining the eyes or gastrointestinal tract. Infections range in severity from asymptomatic to fulminant illnesses with high fever, liver and kidney failure, circulatory collapse, and death. The latter form of the infection, known as "Weil's disease," is named after the German physician who provided one of the first descriptions of the illness in 1886. In patients in whom the bacteria invade the central nervous system (a condition known as "meningoencephalitis"), intense, throbbing headaches are common and are sometimes accompanied by delirium. Thus, Saladin's terminal illness had several features typical of Weil's disease. However, human infections are most common in the late summer and early fall in temperate regions, when temperatures are ideal for growth of the bacteria in the environment. Saladin's illness developed during the winter. Moreover, Beha Ed-din was not a physician and likely used "biliary fever" as a term for fevers in general, rather than to indicate particular illnesses producing both fever and jaundice.

Although typhoid fever, malaria, and typhus also were almost certainly prevalent in medieval Palestine, and no doubt carried off substantial numbers of Christians and Muslims during the Crusades, they were unlikely causes of Saladin's fatal illness. With regard to typhoid, one of many gastrointestinal infections that plagued armies prior to the advent of modern sanitation (see Chapter 3 in *Post Mortem I*), headache is a common early complaint but disorientation is not (33). Moreover, abdominal distress is a prominent feature of the illness, and Saladin apparently had no abdominal pain or tenderness, no nausea or vomiting, and no constipation or diarrhea to support the diagnosis.

Malaria is a more likely possibility in that, like tuberculosis, it commonly induces night sweats (21). Falciparum malaria, caused by the most virulent species of malaria, *Plasmodium falciparum*, can invade the central nervous system to cause fever, headache, disorientation, and death. However, like leptospirosis, it is an infection that tends to disappear during the winter when low temperatures cause its mosquito vector to become less active. Additionally, invasion of the central nervous system by *P. falciparum* occurs predominantly in children. Because of prior exposure to the parasite, adults who survive their initial attack develop partial immunity to the parasite and rarely develop the cerebral form of the infection (34).

Finally, typhus, a bacterial infection transmitted from human to human by body lice, has long been a shadowy companion of war (35). Napoleon's Grand Army was devastated by the infection during his Russian campaign, and during the Great War of 1914–1918 and its aftermath, an estimated 30 million cases of typhus with 3 million deaths occurred in the Soviet Union alone. However, typhus produces a distinctive rash that begins on the trunk and spreads "centrifugally" to the extremities. Saladin had no such rash. What is more, he and his fellow Muslims were "particular about their bathing and beards (36)" and, hence, less prone to infestations by lice than the Franks. For these reasons, of all the possible causes of Saladin's fatal illness, tuberculous meningitis remains the one most consistent with its clinical and epidemiological features.

Beha Ed-din's account of Saladin's final illness has perhaps as much to tell about the nature of medicine in the Sultan's court as about his diagnosis. The "chief physician" to whom Beha Ed-Din refers quite possibly was Maimonides (1135–1204), a Jew who was appointed court physician by Saladin's vizier, Al Fadil, in 1187, 6 years before the Sultan's death (37). Maimonides subsequently became the personal physician of Saladin's eldest son, Al Afdal (38). Like his Arab counterparts, he was a product of the Hippocratic school and an acolyte of Galen. He wrote a famous compendium of medicine in which he endeavored to clarify Galen's interpretation of Hippocratic concepts (39, 40).

Galen, a Greek physician from Pergamum (Turkey) who lived and practiced in the 2nd century AD, did more than any other person to promote the teachings of the "divine Hippocrates." At the time of Galen's birth, Pergamum was a capital of medicine, with a magnificent library and an Asclepieum—a place of worship as well as a renowned medical center that attracted prominent patients and physicians alike. He also studied at the other great medical centers of the ancient world, notably Alexandria, where he completed his medical education, and Rome, where he lived and practiced medicine for over three decades beginning in 162. Through experiments conducted on Barbary apes and fallen gladiators, Galen verified, interpreted, and expanded Hippocratic concepts and then disseminated his interpretations with such energy and skill that they dominated medical thought for over a millennium. As one commentator of the 6th century put it: "Hippocrates sowed, Galen cultivated!" (39).

Although the humoral theory lies at the heart of Hippocratic concepts of health and disease, there was no single such theory to which all Hippocratic physicians subscribed (40). The most widely accepted one maintained that health is determined by a proper balance between four vital humors (blood, phlegm, yellow bile, and black bile), and disease is the consequence of imbalances in these humors (called "dyscrasias"), the specific character of which determines both the nature of the disorder and its treatment (41).

Beha Ed-din's personal belief in the humoral theory is reflected in his comment that "the humors of the body [of Saladin] began to cease their flow" immediately after he was bled. Likewise, the bleeding indicates both a commitment of Saladin's physicians to Hippocratic doctrine and their attribution of the Sultan's illness to a humoral dyscrasia (i.e., a humoral imbalance), which they hoped to alleviate by altering the distribution of the vital humor(s) responsible for the dyscrasia.

Beha Ed-din reported that Saladin's "bilious fever" was "internal rather than external." Hippocratic physicians favored such a binary classification of diseases, separating those due to some internal cause from ones provoked by external factors. Those arising from things inside the body included dyscrasias of bile, phlegm, and the other humors. Those originating from sources outside the body were related to "exertions and wounds, and from heat that makes it too hot, and cold that makes it too cold" (42). As noted above, Beha Ed-din placed Saladin's disorder in the former category.

Saladin was treated with bloodletting, clysters (enemas), and medicines and draughts of unknown composition. In *Disease II* (another of the Hippocratic treatises), the recommended treatment for diseases of the head includes not just three types of evacuants (of which Saladin received only one that we know of) but also no fewer than eight cauterizations of the skull (of which he apparently received none), two beside the ears, two on the temples, two in the back of the head, and two on the nose near the corners of the eyes (43).

With regard to the second form of treatment, Hippocratic physicians used vomiting and bowel evacuations as both preventive and curative measures. Good hygiene was thought to require "that vomiting be induced in winter and bowel evacuation in summer" (44). As explained by the author of *Nature of Man*:

Emetics and clysters for the bowels should be used thus: Use emetics during the six winter months, for this period engenders more phlegm than does the summer, and in it occur the diseases that attack the head and the region above the diaphragm. But when the weather is hot use clysters, for the season is burning, the body bilious, heaviness is felt in the loins and the knees, feverishness comes on and colic in the belly. So the body must be cooled, and the humours that rise must be drawn downwards from these regions. (44)

Saladin's disease of the head was treated with clysters in late February—the dead of winter. Moreover, the clysters were administered on the tenth day of his illness, when he was clearly moribund, which was contrary to one of the fundamental precepts of Hippocratic doctrine—a prohibition against treating patients judged to be incurable (45). Thus, in two respects, the physicians who treated Saladin during his final illness appear to have violated Hippocratic standards of practice.

Hippocratic physicians were ambivalent about medicines. *Pharmacopoles*, the forerunners of modern pharmacists, sold both poisons and medicines under the ambiguous title of *pharmakon*, suggesting that the disciples of Hippocrates were as cognizant as their modern counterparts of the capacity of drugs to harm patients as well as to help them (46). Although the specific medications used to treat Saladin are unknown, it's likely that they were dictated by the "Doctrine of the Signatures," then in vogue in the Levant (47). According to the doctrine, the way plants (and presumably animals and minerals) look, feel, taste, or react dictates their proper clinical application. Treatments were based on similarities between therapeutic substances used and the diseased human organs, correlation between the color of the substance and the color of the patient, similarities between the substance and the patient's symptoms, and the use of substances that might produce symptoms of particular diseases in healthy persons to remedy those same symptoms in those who were sick. The shape of a walnut seed, for example, which has features similar to that of the human brain, was "favored as a treatment for clearing and curing the brain during the Middle Ages."

When Saladin's counter-crusade was over and his eyes closed in death, he was so poor there was not even enough of the vast wealth he had conquered left to pay for his funeral. So irresistible had been his impulse for giving that "in his treasury there remained only one Tyrian gold piece and forty-seven pieces of silver" (48). None of his 17 sons inherited Saladin's generosity or statesmanship. Shortly after their father's death they began fighting amongst themselves, and in just a few years had reduced his empire (Fig. 4.2) to a fragmented pastiche of powerless states.

Beha Ed-din outlived his master long enough to see Jerusalem return to the Franks, as Saladin had feared. Emperor Frederick II negotiated its surrender with Saladin's nephew, al-Kamil, in 1229. (49). Had the Sultan not succumbed to his final illness but lived a while longer, it's not likely that the course of history would have been different, for "evil old age that comes to all" (50) was already heavy upon him.

Richard (Fig. 4.3) recovered from the illness for which Saladin sent him fruit and snow and embarked upon an odyssey that became the principal substance of the Lionheart legend. Six months after leaving the Palestinian city of Acre by ship with a band of close confederates, he landed in Corfu. No longer a hero, he was hunted throughout Europe by legions of enemies inflamed by a series of slanderous accusations spread by Philip Augustus. The Duke of Austria, in particular, was eager to apprehend him for having dragged his treasured banner through the dust after the fall of Acre during the recent Crusade.

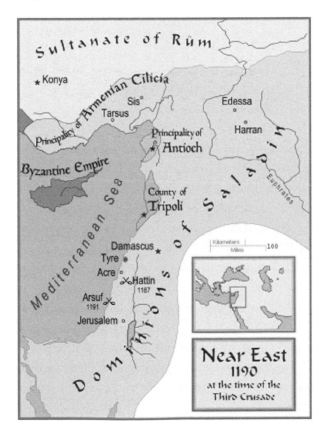

FIGURE 4.2 Map of the Near East in 1190 AD, showing Saladin's dominions 3 years before his death. (From Shepherd WR [1911]. *Europe and the Mediterranean Lands about 1190*. Available online at http://www.lib.utexas.edu/maps/historical/shepherd_1911/shepherd-c-070–071.jpg.)

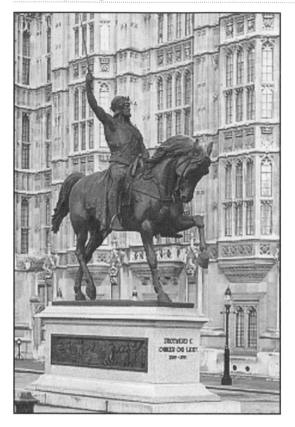
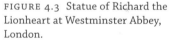

FIGURE 4.3 Statue of Richard the Lionheart at Westminster Abbey, London.

Richard next traveled in secret to Ragusa (Dubrovnik) and then Aquileia, north of Trieste, after having been shipwrecked, then from Friuli through the Alps into Carinthia, all the while pursued by his enemies. When he reached the outskirts of Vienna, he was finally taken prisoner by his arch-enemy, Leopold, Duke of Austria, who had him escorted west along the Danube to imprisonment in the towering castle of Dürnstein. In February 1193, Richard was sold to the Holy Roman Emperor, Henry VI, for 60,000 pounds of silver. The transaction gave the emperor an opportunity to avenge Richard's role in the loss of Sicily from the Holy Roman Empire. It also led to the excommunication of Leopold for having imprisoned a royal pilgrim and having received "Judas silver" in his deal with Henry VI.

Richard remained Henry's prisoner until February 4, 1194, when a ransom of 70,000 marks of silver was finally raised. His mother, Eleanor of Aquitaine, played a pivotal role in his release, having pled her son's case with passion and veiled threats throughout his imprisonment.

Richard wasted little time in settling scores with his former lover, Philip Augustus, and brother, Earl John, who had sliced away his domain in his absence. He set foot on English soil at Sandwich on March 12 and by Easter time was crowned Richard I of England a second time. Within a week he left England for Normandy and a protracted campaign against Philip. The first year alone, he reclaimed his castles at Vermeuil, Loches, and Montmirail, besting Philip whenever the two monarchs came into direct combat. After an uncertain truce through 1196–97, war resumed more violently than ever. However, this time the Pope intervened, and Richard reluctantly agreed to a treaty of 5 years. But Richard loved war, and when his accounts with Philip were finally settled, he sought new excuses for combat. The viscount of a castle in Limoges gave him one by withholding a portion of a treasure Richard considered his due. In the punitive siege that resulted, Richard was wounded by a young crossbowman while strutting before the walls of the beleaguered citadel without his armor. The shaft of the arrow was removed promptly from his arm, but not the metal tip. When finally the tip was removed, the arm was blackened with gangrene. Richard ordered all of the defenders of the castle hanged, save the young bowman, Peter Basil, who had shot him. When the boy was dragged before him, he demanded: "What harm have I done you that you have killed me?" When the boy answered that the king had killed his father and two brothers and intended to kill him as well, Richard reportedly forgave him and had him presented with 100 shillings English and released. Richard died on April 6, 1199, "a lion slain by an ant" (23).

References

1. Herschel AJ. *Maimonides* (translated from German by Neugroschell J). Toronto: McGraw-Hill Ryerson Ltd, 1982:51.

2. Reston J Jr. *Warriors of God. Richard the Lionheart and Saladin in the Third Crusade.* New York: Anchor Books, 2001:9–17.

3. Rosebault CJ. *Saladin. Prince of Chivalry.* New York: Robert M. McBride & Co., 1930:194–196.

4. Newby PH. *Saladin in His Time.* New York: Dorset Press, 1983:39.

5. Ibid., p. 199.

6. Ibid., pp. 30, 79, 80.

7. Ibid., p. 29.

8. Ibid., p. 14.

9. Op. cit. Rosebault, p. 62.

10. Op. cit. Newby, p. 50.

11. Ibid., pp. 53, 115–135.

12. Ibid., p. 102.

13. Beha E-D. *The Life of Saladin.* London: Committee of the Palestine Exploration Fund, 1897:1–409.

14. Ibid., p. 102.

15. Op. cit. Newby, pp. 21–25.

16. Ibid., p. 105.

17. Ibid., p. 130.

18. Op. cit. Beha, p. 193.

19. Ibid., pp. 217–219.

20. Ibid,. p. 229.

21. Fairhurst RM, Wellems TE. Plasmodium species (malaria). In Mandell GL, Bennett JE, Dolin R, eds. *Principles and Practice of Infectious Diseases*, 7th ed. Philadelphia: Churchill Livingstone Elsevier, 2010:3437–3462.

22. Op. cit. Newby, p. 65.

23. Op. cit. Reston, pp. 338–346, 358–383.

24. Op. cit. Beha, p. 379.

25. Ibid., p. 304.

26. Op. cit. Newby, p. 158.

27. Ibid., p. 181.

28. Op. cit. Beha, pp. 400–406.

29. Op. cit. Reston, pp. 356–357.

30. Dubos R, Dubos J. *The White Plague. Tuberculosis, Man and Society*. Boston: Little, Brown and Co., 1952:6, 7.

31. Dormandy T. *The White Death. A History of Tuberculosis*. New York: New York University Press, 2000:4, 5.

32. Levett PN, Haake DA. Leptospira species (leptospirosis). In Mandell GL, Bennett JE, Dolin R, eds. *Principles and Practice of Infectious Diseases*, 7th ed. Philadelphia: Churchill Livingstone Elsevier, 2010:3059–3065.

33. Thielman NM, Crump JA, Guerrant RL. Enteric fever and other causes of abdominal symptoms with fever. In Mandell GL, Bennett JE, Dolin R, eds. *Principles and Practice of Infectious Diseases*, 7th ed. Philadelphia: Churchill Livingstone Elsevier, 2010:1399–1412.

34. Roth H. 100 Cases of Cerebral Malaria. *E African Med J* 1956;33:405–407.

35. Walker DH, Raoult D. *Rickettsia prowazekii* (epidemic or louse-borne typhus). In Mandell GL, Bennett JE, Dolin R, eds. *Principles and Practice of Infectious Diseases*, 7th ed. Philadelphia: Churchill Livingstone Elsevier, 2010:2521–2524.

36. Op. cit. Rosebault, p. 128.

37. Op. cit. Herschel, p. 182.

38. Ibid., p. 233.

39. Ibid., pp. 213–215.

40. Jouanna J. *Hippocrates* (translated by MB DeBevoisse). Baltimore: Johns Hopkins University Press, 1999:316, 353–357.

41. Ibid., pp. 325–327.

42. Ibid., p. 146.

43. Ibid., p. 161.

44. Ibid., p. 156.

45. Ibid., p. 107.

46. Ibid., p. 130.

47. Lev E. The doctrine of signatures in the Medieval and Ottoman Levant. *Vesalius* 2002;8:13–22.

48. Op. cit. Rosebault, p. 173.

49. Op. cit. Newby, p. 198.

50. Homer. *The Iliad* (translated by E. Rees). New York: Barnes and Noble Classics, 2005:65.

5 "Interred at the Least Possible Expense"

IN 1805, NAPOLEON, musing gloomily over the news from Trafalgar, asked Berthier, his Minister of War: "How old was [this patient] when he died?" Berthier replied that he thought he was 45 years old. "Then," said Napoleon, "he did not fulfill his destiny. Had he lived to this time, France might have had an Admiral" (1).

Twenty-six years earlier, when Richard Pearson, captain of the HMS *Serapis*, finally shouted: "Sir I have struck! I ask for quarter!," this same patient became the first captain of an American Navy ship to defeat and capture a British man-of-war of any real size or strength (2). The crowd of over a thousand people gathered atop the cliffs of Flamborough Head on England's east coast to watch their ship of the line trap and destroy the American pirate was stunned (3). The patient's ship was old and slow with obsolete cannon of dubious reliability. The *Serapis* was faster, heavily armed, and brand new. Moreover, it was manned by a crew buoyed by a centuries-old tradition of British naval supremacy (4).

However, this patient was no ordinary sea wolf. On the rebel side, the story of the American War of Independence at sea was largely one of bumbling incompetence. This captain was a powerful exception—a strategist and a commander well ahead of his time. He was intrepid, unprincipled, reckless, predatory, and ambitious, and though civilized in externals, he was savage at heart (5). Mortal peril invigorated him, made him more nimble and clever (6). He was also uncommonly lucky.

Most sea captains of the era adhered to an unwritten code that allowed them to break off an engagement before it devolved into senseless slaughter, but not this one. He fought to the death with an all-out pursuit of victory, no matter the odds, no matter the cost, that was a harbinger of today's total war (7). In his battle with the *Serapis*, the carnage on both ships was unspeakable. When it finally ended, the *Serapis* was on fire. The *Bonhomme Richard*, his ship, was so badly mauled by the *Serapis*, in addition to friendly fire from the *Alliance*, she succumbed to her mortal wounds the very next day and plunged bow first into the sea, her American colors waving defiantly till the last (8).

This patient's contributions to the success of the American fight for independence were such that Thomas Jefferson was moved to write: "I consider this officer to be the principal hope of our future efforts on the ocean." At Monticello, he displayed the patient's bust alongside those of Washington, Franklin, and Lafayette (9).

In November 1777, it was this patient, in command of the *Ranger*, who carried dispatches to France announcing the American victory over General Burgoyne that helped draw France as an ally into the war (10). He was befriended by Benjamin Franklin, then minister to France, in whose honor he named his most famous ship the *Bonhomme Richard* (after "Poor Richard" of Franklin's almanac).

In April 1778, he entered the Firth of Solway, his old home waters, and invaded Whitehaven to show the British that the American War of Independence was not some far-off colonial dust-up but a threat to their own livelihoods and security. It had been more than 700 years since England had been invaded by a foreign power (11).

He then sailed 20 miles across the Firth for St. Mary's Isle, where he hoped to find and kidnap the Earl of Selkirk so that he might be traded for imprisoned Continental Navy sailors. Unfortunately, the Earl was absent and not taken. Nevertheless, the psychological impact of the raids was considerable. They terrorized the civilian population to such an extent that Britain's Secretary of State was moved to declare: "The rebel privateer which plundered Lord Selkirk's house has thrown the whole western coast into consternation" (12). The raids also so blackened the patient's name that never again could he return to his ancestral home (13).

Three men-of-war were dispatched to the area in search of the elusive privateer. They never found him. However, he found one of theirs, the *Drake*, a 20-gun sloop-of-war. Though his men were untested and lacked the other side's sense of invincibility, training, or discipline, he outsmarted his opponent in what was another first—a ship of the American navy defeating a comparable British warship in one-on-one combat (10).

He was a fearsome commander but not without flaws. He was "leprous with vanity" (14). His ambition, which was limitless, ever-present, and all-consuming, was a source of strength but also a vice. He was insecure, exalting in moments of battle but then prone to brooding in the aftermath. Usually mild and soft-spoken, he was also fussy and quick-tempered. These were the traits that later would make him less of an admiral than a ship's captain.

He was a visionary. When the American War of Independence had been won, he imagined his adopted country as a mighty sea power before it had either the capacity or the will to become one. He pleaded with the new nation to empower him to build a navy to rival those of Great Britain and France, one that could protect the country's commercial and security interests at sea (15). His proposal was brushed off, as was he. The new nation had no further use for him. When he died in Paris in 1792 of a mysterious illness at the age of 45, lonely and forgotten, the American minister's only interest in him was that his remains "be interred in the most private manner and at the least possible expense" (16). Fortunately for posterity, and the investigation into the cause of the patient's death, the French government had the foresight to bury the American naval hero submerged in alcohol in a lead coffin in the event that a more enlightened American government one day would wish to reclaim and properly honor him (16).

The patient's early years offer no clue as to the cause of the mysterious illness that would take his life. He was born on July 6, 1747, on the 1,500-acre estate of Arbigland that rims the Firth of Solway in western Scotland. His father was a gardener. His mother kept house for William Craik, the master of the estate. They had seven children, four boys and three girls. The two youngest boys died in infancy and the eldest girl died in her teens, all of unknown cause. The eldest son, William, was adopted by a Virginia planter, William Jones, who had taken a liking to the boy during a visit to his former home in Scotland (10, 17).

Almost from the first, the patient seemed bred to the sea. As a child, he watched the great ships slipping down the Firth of Solway to the Irish Sea and beyond, and dreamt of joining the Royal Navy. However, being of modest parentage, he lacked the social connections necessary to obtain a midshipman's berth and had to settle for a position as an ordinary seaman aboard a merchantman. He was 13 when he went to sea for the first time aboard the *Friendship*, a two-masted brig out of Whitehaven, just across the Firth of Solway. For three years he crisscrossed the Atlantic on the *Friendship*, sustained on an unvarying diet of pickled beef, dried peas, and weevil biscuits. These he washed down with lemon or lime juice and sugar mixed with water. He never developed a taste for grog, only wine, of which, in later life, he consumed "three glasses after dinner in good weather" (18).

In 1764, after having crossed the Atlantic eight times, he was released from his apprenticeship aboard the *Friendship* and took a wretched position as third mate aboard a slaver, the *King George*, also out of Whitehaven. After two years, he transferred to another "blackbirder," the *Two Friends*, as first mate. When he had sailed the infamous "middle passage" between Africa and the slave plantations of the Caribbean for another two years, he had had enough and asked to be paid off. Unemployed and in Kingston, he obtained free passage home aboard a brig, the

John. Both the captain and the first mate died of "tropical fever" during the voyage, leaving the patient as the only man on board capable of navigating the ship. When he brought the *John* home safely, the owners rewarded him with command of the vessel (19). He was 21, master of his first ship and yet to suffer any serious illness.

His first illness of note occurred when he was 26. At the time, he was making his way from London to the West Indies with a load of butter and wine as master of the *Betsy.* During a layover in Ireland to repair the ship's frame, he developed a "severe fever" that sent him to bed for 16 days and left him "much reduced." Nothing more is known of the illness other than he recovered fully, set sail two months later with a new cargo (the butter had spoiled), and arrived in Tobago just before Christmas 1773. There he killed the ringleader of an attempted mutiny in self-defense. Rather than face a potentially hostile jury of the victim's hometown in a local court, he decided to flee to the American continent until able to stand trial at some later date before an Admiralty Court (20).

He then disappeared from the historical record for two years before resurfacing with a new name in Fredericksburg, Virginia, at his brother's plantation. His brother was mortally ill and died of an unknown disease shortly after the patient arrived. Following the funeral, the patient managed his brother's estate and briefly considered becoming a planter himself. However, the American Revolution was brewing, and in 1775, he answered a call from the Congressional Marine Committee to help develop plans for a Continental Navy (10).

On December 7, 1775, he was commissioned as a first lieutenant in the Continental Navy (21). He spent the next eight years on the quarterdeck of fighting ships plowing the sea for the American cause. Many of his men paid the butcher's bill for his mad quest for glory during those years. Incredibly, he was never wounded himself (22). During one voyage, a member of his crew came down with smallpox (23). Other diseases likely were also prevalent aboard his ships. However, except for chronic insomnia (24), the patient's health remained robust until July 1779, when he had a brief unspecified illness shortly before his historic battle with the *Serapis* (25).

In February 1780, he was again sick, this time "blind with sore eyes, which [prevented him]...from paying a visit to...friends on shore." He was much agitated, biting his lips often and walking the quarterdeck muttering to himself. He acted "Queeg-like, suspicious, jumpy and slightly dotty" and complained of feeling old, though he was only 33. He wondered if his warrior days were coming to an end (26).

He soon recovered and sailed to Paris, where he was "feasted and caressed by all the world" for his stunning exploits against the Royal Navy. Pursued by women of all classes, he promptly began sailing the obscene waves of torrid affairs involving myriad women ranging from prostitutes to grand dames. He was "a callous lover, even measured by the mores of his times" (27).

After the cessation of hostilities between Britain and her former colonies in April 1783, the patient returned to America, where "recurring tropical fever" again troubled him. He was too sick to participate in the courts martial of two captains who had lost their ships during the war. He traveled to the mountains of Pennsylvania, where he "took the cure" at a retreat near the town of Bethlehem. Nothing more is known of the character of his illness or its treatment, other than he again appears to have recovered completely (28).

With the war ended, the patient was restless and frustrated. When the Continental Congress refused his offer to build the new nation's navy, he turned to Thomas Jefferson for help in returning to duty so that he might again pursue glory at sea. Jefferson advised him to contact Catherine, Tsarina of Russia, who he had recently learned was interested in having the patient command her Black Sea fleet in a campaign to liberate Constantinople from the Ottoman Turks. Though 40 years old, no longer in the best of health, and having not commanded a ship of war at sea for more than eight years, the patient accepted an offer from Catherine the Great to become an admiral in the Russian Navy (29).

He left Paris for Copenhagen in late winter, arriving in the Danish court shivering and exhausted with symptoms of a lung infection. He wrote Jefferson to say: "My suffering, from the inclemency of the weather and my want of proper means to guard against it on the journey, were inexpressible; and I believe, from what I feel will continue to affect my constitution." He pushed on to Stockholm and then across the Gulfs of Bothnia and Finland under appalling conditions, finally reaching a still-frozen St. Petersburg the first week of May 1787 (30).

He took command of the Black Sea fleet in late May. In June, he met the Turkish armada at the Liman (the estuary where the Dnieper and Bug Rivers empty into the Black Sea) and defeated it in two decisive engagements. Whether he deserved credit for the victories, or his Russian counterpart, depends on whose accounts of the battles one chooses to believe. Catherine believed her Russian admiral, Prince Nassau-Siegen, deserved the credit and rewarded him generously. She recognized the efforts of her American admiral with only a minor medal, the Order of St. Anne, and a meaningless appointment as commander of her idle Northern Fleet. While traveling north along the Dnieper to assume his new command, the patient again became desperately ill with symptoms of pneumonia (31).

In September 1789, the patient left Russia in disgrace after having been accused of raping a 10 year old German girl. Eventually, the girl's mother admitted that she had been given money by "a man with decorations" in return for a damaging story about the patient. However, by then, enemies in the Russian court had succeeded in destroying the foreign admiral. For all practical purposes, the patient, now in a suicidal state, was finished in the Russian Navy. He asked for and was granted a two-year leave of absence, which allowed him to retain his pay and emoluments, and left Russia, never to return (32).

He drifted from Poland to Austria and then to Holland and Britain, all the while struggling against the headwinds of deteriorating health, before finally reaching Paris in May 1789. He had a hacking cough and appeared gray and fatigued. According to the English writer Thomas Carlyle, he looked "like a ghost of himself." He had trouble speaking, and when he did speak, he was barely audible. He felt betrayed and floated into a deepening gloom (33).

Shortly before his 45th birthday, his health declined precipitously. His close friend, Col. Samuel Blackden, gave the following vivid account of the patient's final days:

> But for two months past he began to lose his appetite, grew yellow, and showed symptoms of jaundice. For this he took medical treatment and for a short time seemed to grow better. A few days before his death his legs began to swell, which proceeded upward to his body, so that for two days before his decease he could not button his waistcoat and had great difficulty in breathing.... [He] put off the making of his will until the afternoon of July 18 [1792], when he was prevailed upon to send for a notary and made his will. M. Beaupoil and myself witnessed it and left him sitting in a chair in his parlor. A few minutes after we retired he walked into his chamber and laid himself upon his face on the bedside, with his feet on the floor. The Queen's physician, who was attending him, came soon after, and on entering the apartment found him in that position, and on trying to lift him up found that he had expired. His disorder had terminated in dropsy of the heart. His body was put into a leaden coffin on the 20th, that, in case the United States, which he had so essentially served and with so much honor, should claim his remains they might be more easily removed. (16)

For John Paul Jones (né John Paul) (Fig. 5.1), the ever-flowing stream of time had run dry. Gone was a man to match the sea.

If this were all we knew of John Paul Jones' medical condition, we would have no hope of diagnosing his fatal disorder. But fortunately we also have the results of an autopsy—albeit one performed 113 years after his death.

In 1899, more than a century after Jones was buried, former Union Army Brig. General Horace Porter, who was then the American ambassador to France, began a search for the Revolutionary hero's remains. On review of Jones' certificate of burial, Porter succeeded in identifying the site of interment as the cemetery of St. Louis "for foreign Protestants" in the northeastern section of Paris. Urban sprawl had long since

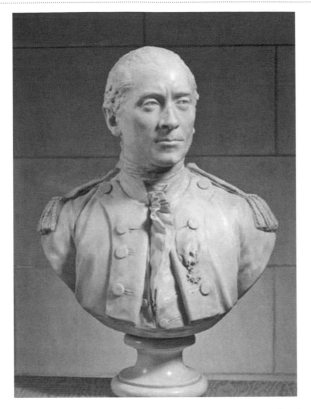

FIGURE 5.1 White marble bust of John Paul Jones by Jean-Antoine Houdon (1747–1792) dated 1781 and generally regarded as the most accurate likeness of the subject. (With permission from the U.S. Naval Academy Museum, Annapolis, MD)

overrun the abandoned cemetery, which was covered almost completely with buildings of an inferior class. After securing the rights to excavate the site in 1905, Porter began probing it with shafts and tunnels at his own expense, ultimately uncovering five lead coffins, three of which bore copper plates inscribed with names other than "Jones" and a fourth containing a skeleton measuring 6'2" in length (16).

When the team opened the fifth coffin, they found a well-preserved body (Fig. 5.2), evidently originally submerged in alcohol, which had long since evaporated. It was wrapped in a linen shroud "bearing a small initial worked with thread, either a 'J' or, if read upside down, a 'P'." The body was transported to the Paris School of Medicine, where Dr. J. Capitan and Dr. G. Papillault, two renowned professors of anthropology, performed a thorough scientific examination. They verified beyond any reasonable doubt that the body was that of Admiral John Paul Jones by means of "measurements [i.e., height (5'7"), hair color, a distinctive earlobe, absence of wounds, and facial features corresponding perfectly with those of the Houdon bust of the admiral], the autopsy [see below], marks upon the linen;

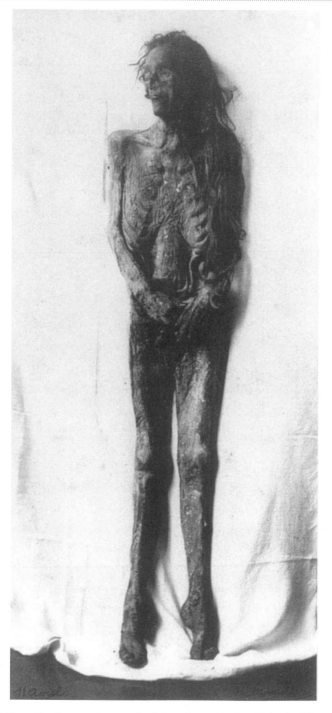

FIGURE 5.2 F. Monpillard's 1905 photograph of the exhumed body of John Paul Jones. (With permission from the U.S. Naval Historical Center, Washington, DC)

[and]...that the body had been carefully preserved and packed as if to prepare it for a long voyage...in case the United States...should claim his remains" (34).

The autopsy, performed by Capitan and Dr. Victor Cornil, revealed the following:

"The only organs which were injured were the kidneys [Fig. 5.3]. As far as can be judged, by examination of the badly preserved viscera [including the heart, aorta, liver, gallbladder, and spleen but not the brain], we believe that the case in point is interstitial nephritis, with fibrous degeneracy of the glomeruli of Malpighi, which quite agrees with the symptoms observed during life (34)...Sections of [the liver], slightly magnified, resembled perfectly those of a normal liver...[The kidneys] revealed glomerulose lesions...real interstitial glomerulitis far advanced on some glomeruli thus transformed into fibrous nodules. Moreover, the Bowman capsules were at times much thickened. The arteries were likewise very thick and surrounded or filled with crystals of fat." (35)

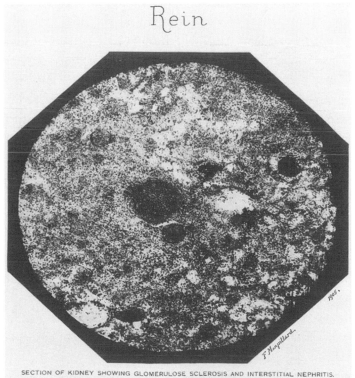

SECTION OF KIDNEY SHOWING GLOMERULOSE SCLEROSIS AND INTERSTITIAL NEPHRITIS.
(Enlarged 100 diameters.)

FIGURE 5.3 Section of John Paul Jones' kidney prepared by Prof. Cornil and purportedly showing fibrosis of the glomeruli and interstitial nephritis (original magnification ×100). (With permission from the U.S. Naval Historical Center, Washington, DC)

A search for tubercle bacilli (the bacteria responsible for tuberculosis) in the lungs was negative. Only a small area of healed pneumonia surrounded by fibrous tissue was identified in the left lung (4).

Even given the results of the autopsy, what we know of John Paul Jones' medical history does not permit a definitive diagnosis of any of his illnesses. Although grossly the body was surprisingly well preserved after 113 years, the cellular structure of its various organs was not. Thus, whereas the autopsy clearly incriminated the kidneys as the seat of Jones' final (fatal) illness, it failed to identify the specific disorder that destroyed them. Nevertheless, Jones' clinical record and post-mortem examination do provide enough details of the nature of his various illnesses to narrow the list of possible causes to just a few (36).

With regard to the series of illnesses that afflicted him between 1770 and 1783, most appear to have been infections contracted during service in the West Indies or possibly as a result of his intemperate sex life. Dengue (a mosquito-borne viral infection) or malaria would have been the most likely etiology of his severe and protracted illnesses during this period. Dengue is an especially attractive diagnosis for the illness of 1780, in that it is commonly associated with intense eye pain (which might explain Jones' "eyes so sore he was almost blind"), as well as marked fatigue, and muscle and joint pains (which could have accounted for his feeling "like an old man" though only in his thirties) (37). Leptospirosis (a systemic infection caused by a corkscrew-shaped bacterium acquired from rodents and sometimes other animals) is another diagnosis worth considering as the cause of that illness, both because it is commonly accompanied by inflammation of the eyelids (conjunctivitis), which might explain the eye complaints, and also inflammation of the brain (meningoencephalitis), which might have been the reason for Jones' "Queeg-like" behavior during the illness (38).

With regard to sexually transmitted diseases—syphilis in particular—there is no doubt that John Paul Jones was at considerable risk for such infections. The prevalence of syphilis among the general population in both Europe and America during his lifetime likely exceeded 10%. Moreover, syphilis increases in frequency during times of war and is most prevalent among prostitutes and their clients (39). The extent of Jones' philandering (and hence his risk of having contracted syphilis) was apparently extraordinary, even by naval standards of his era (27). Nevertheless, neither his clinical history nor his autopsy findings show evidence of this infection.

The pulmonary problems that developed at the age of 41 during Jones' grueling journey to St. Petersburg were almost certainly manifestations of bacterial pneumonia. Both his symptoms at that time and the results of his post-mortem examination favor this diagnosis.

All of the illnesses that preceded Jones' final one seem to have resolved without long-term sequelae. It is, nevertheless, possible that they planted the immunological seed that later flowered into his fatal kidney disorder. His pneumonia, for example, might have done so, in that proliferative glomerulonephritis (inflammation of the glomeruli—the microscopic filters within the kidneys) (Fig. 5.4) sometimes develops as a consequence of a host of infections, including those caused by the pneumococcus (40), *Klebsiella* (41), *Mycoplasma* (42), influenza, and adenovirus (43, 44). However, such associated renal abnormalities are rare and have not been shown to progress to end-stage kidney disease.

On post-mortem examination, "the only organs that were injured were the kidneys... [which were]... small, hard and contracted" (16). Because the liver was "normal, with its anatomical disposition very clear" (16), Jones' terminal ascites and peripheral edema are explained better by advanced renal failure, possibly complicated by the nephrotic syndrome (Mozart's fatal disorder; see Chapter 8 in *Post Mortem I* (45)), than by hepatic failure. Likewise, because the liver was apparently normal, the terminal "jaundice" reported by Col. Blackden was more likely due to florid uremia (accumulation of massive amounts of waste

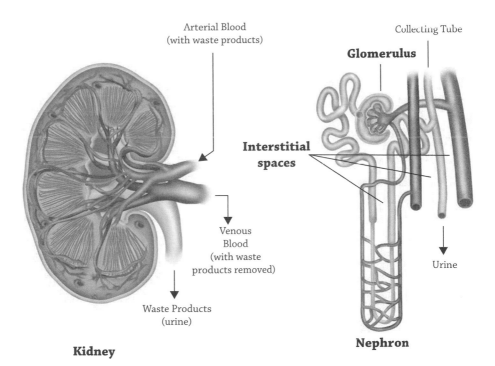

FIGURE 5.4 Diagram of the human kidney, showing the basic structure of the nephron, many thousands of which filter waste products from the blood and process them into urine. Note the glomerulus (the kidney's micro-filter) and the interstitial spaces, which are composed of support tissue and become infiltrated by inflammatory cells during "interstitial nephritis."

products within the body), during which accumulation of carotene-like pigments combined with anemia gives the skin a yellow cast (46), rather than due to high levels of bilirubin in the blood (hyperbilirubinemia) due to poor liver function. If Jones was as uremic as these findings suggest, his precipitous demise likely would have been the consequence of a cardiac arrhythmia or some other fatal complication of uremia.

Based on the microscopic examination of the kidneys, Professor Cornil diagnosed both "interstitial nephritis" and "interstitial glomerulitis" (two inflammatory disorders of the kidney in which the inflammation is located primarily in the interstitium) (Fig. 5.4) (16). Thus, what he appears to have seen in the microscopic sections of Jones' kidneys, which have since been lost, was generalized "interstitial inflammation," which can be seen in the advanced stages of both chronic interstitial nephritis and glomerulonephritis.

If the Admiral's fatal kidney disorder was chronic interstitial nephritis, as has been espoused since his autopsy in 1905 (10, 16, 47), the question remains as to its cause. Today urinary obstruction (due to problems such as kidney stones or an enlarged prostate), urinary reflux (i.e., urinary backflow), analgesics (e.g., ibuprofen and the other nonsteroidal anti-inflammatory drugs), heavy metals, and hardening of the small arteries of the kidneys (arteriolar nephrosclerosis) are the principal causes of chronic interstitial nephritis (48). Because Jones' renal arterioles appeared "very thick" at post-mortem examination (16), arteriolar nephrosclerosis is worth considering as a condition that might have resulted in chronic interstitial nephritis. The absence of obvious left ventricular hypertrophy, however, argues against this diagnosis, since "sustained significant hypertension" (an important cause of left ventricular hypertrophy) is both the hallmark of the disorder and the mechanism by which it produces diffuse tubulointerstitial damage (48).

Given the lack of a history of analgesic abuse and the absence of kidney stones (nephrolithiasis) and urinary anatomical abnormalities on post-mortem examination, the only other cause of chronic interstitial nephritis worth considering is heavy metal intoxication. Of such metals, lead is the one to which Jones most likely would have been exposed. Chronic lead intoxication, in fact, was epidemic in 18th-century Europe, owing to, among other things, the widespread use of lead as a preservative in wine (49). Jones consumed wine sparingly. Moreover, he had none of the other manifestations of chronic lead intoxication, such as chronic constipation, recurrent abdominal pain, or peripheral neuropathy (e.g., focal weakness or paralysis).

Because the principal causes of renal failure in the 18th century might have been different from those of the present, care must be taken in extrapolating current experience to patients of that era. This caveat notwithstanding, glomerulonephritis is at present substantially more common than interstitial nephritis. This fact, combined with Jones' peripheral edema and ascites (which raise the possibility of the nephrotic syndrome), and the absence of an obvious risk factor for interstitial nephritis render this diagnosis less likely than a chronic glomerular disorder.

In clinical practice today, the most common glomerular disorder of adults is IgA nephropathy (kidney disease caused by abnormal deposition of IgA antibodies in kidney tissues), followed by membranous nephropathy, focal segmental glomerulosclerosis, and diabetes. Recently reported histological evidence of IgA nephropathy in Crown Prince Joseph Habsburg, who died in 1847 (50), confirms the existence of the disorder in premodern times but unfortunately tells us nothing about its prevalence in Jones' lifetime. If its relative importance as a cause of progressive glomerular disease has remained constant over the past 200 years, IgA nephropathy would be Jones' most likely diagnosis, based solely on its current relative frequency. Nevertheless, given the histological abnormalities described by Cornil (16), membranous glomerulonephritis, focal segmental glomerulosclerosis, or membranoproliferative glomerulonephritis also could have destroyed the Admiral's kidneys. The absence of a history of recurrent bouts of hematuria (bloody urine) argues against IgA nephropathy but might simply reflect the limitations of Jones' clinical record.

IgA nephropathy is currently the most common form of primary glomerulonephritis worldwide. Although initially considered a benign condition, it is now recognized as a disorder that frequently progresses to renal failure. Its cause is unknown. Infections (such as those to which Jones was exposed throughout his life) and environmental agents have long been suspected of inducing the immunological process responsible for IgA nephropathy. However, no such trigger has yet been identified. A wide variety of kidney lesions have been encountered on light microscopy, including abnormal capillary proliferation, segmental sclerosis, segmental necrosis, and cellular crescent formation. In addition to the glomerular alterations, a variety of nonspecific tubulointerstitial and vascular changes can be seen, including interstitial fibrosis, tubular atrophy, interstitial inflammation, and vascular sclerosis (51). Recent observations suggest that binding of immune complexes (clumps of antibodies) containing aberrantly glycosylated IgA1 to mesangial cells is responsible for these pathological alterations (52).

The official movement to recognize Jones as father of the U.S. Navy began in 1900 when Augustus C. Buell published a two-volume biography entitled *Paul Jones: Founder of the American Navy* (53). Buell, an engineer turned historian, rewrote some of Jones' letters and completely fabricated other documents in promoting him as the father of the U.S. Navy. Critics were suspicious of Buell's documentation and questioned the popular historian's contention that Jones had been a paragon of patriotism and professionalism (54). In spite of the controversy, in 1904, a year after Buell's death, President Theodore Roosevelt publicly endorsed Jones as "Father of the Navy" after Porter located his corpse in the abandoned Parisian cemetery (55).

With the discovery of the naval hero's remains, Roosevelt, who had once dismissed Jones as merely a "daring corsair," now enthusiastically embraced Buell's interpretation of the Jones legend as part of his publicity campaign to build a massive fleet of capital warships staffed by a modern officer corps. Enshrining Jones as father of the Navy gave the President a national hero on whom to focus the country's attention while advocating the importance of a powerful navy to America's role as an emerging world power (56).

Public excitement surrounding Porter's discovery was both instantaneous and impassioned, as the President, State Department, and Navy began planning the largest naval commemoration in American history to honor the once-lost-but-now-found father of the Navy. A far cry from his first funeral, the year-long commemoration began in France on the anniversary of Jones' birth with an impressive memorial service at the American Church of the Holy Trinity. When the squadron carrying the Admiral's remains arrived at Annapolis 13 days later, the U.S. Naval Academy held a brief but dignified service before French and American pallbearers placed the casket in a temporary brick vault to await an elaborate commemorative ceremony scheduled for the following spring (1). However, it was not until 1913 that Congress finally appropriated the funds necessary to complete construction of a permanent resting place for the celebrated corpse—an ornate marble mausoleum reminiscent of Napoleon's (Fig. 5.5) in the basement of the Naval Academy chapel.

So who is the father of the U.S. Navy? John Paul Jones, who once wrote "my desire for fame is infinite," certainly would have welcomed the title. The U.S. Navy, however, believes the honor is more appropriately shared. Its current official position is that because many "played prominent roles in the founding of a national navy . . . the Navy recognizes no one individual as 'Father' to the exclusion of all others . . . The various attempts to credit individual naval officers with this act are misguided." Jones should be remembered in the Navy, according to the Naval Historical Center, "for his indomitable will, his unwillingness to consider surrender when the slightest hope of victory still burned. Throughout his naval career Jones promoted professional standards and training. Sailors of the United States Navy can do no better than to emulate the spirit behind John Paul Jones' stirring declaration: 'I wish to have no connection with any ship that does not sail fast, for I intend to go in harm's way'" (57).

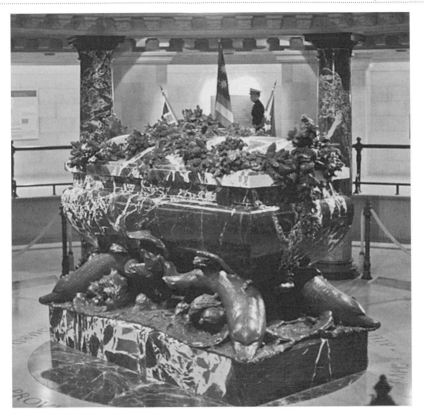

FIGURE 5.5 Tomb of John Paul Jones beneath the U.S. Naval Academy chapel rotunda. Photograph taken at the USNA commencement 2006. (With permission from the U.S. Naval Academy, Annapolis, MD)

References

1. Marion H. *John Paul Jones' Last Cruise and Final Resting Place: The United States Naval Academy*. Washington, DC: George E. Howard, 1906:11.

2. Thomas E. *John Paul Jones. Sailor, Hero, Father of the American Navy*. New York: Simon & Schuster, 2003:194.

3. Ibid., p. 189.

4. Ibid., p. 1, 2.

5. Ibid., p. 6.

6. Ibid., p. 60.

7. Ibid., p. 8.

8. Ibid., p. 178–198.

9. Ibid., p. 7.

10. Vincent EH. Death comes for the admiral. *Surg Gynecol Obstet* 1949;89:779–783.

11. Op. cit. Thomas, p. 117.

12. Ibid., p. 133.

13. Ibid., p. 128.

14. Ibid., p. 10.

15. Ibid., p. 5.

16. Porter H, Vignaud H. Gowdy JK, et al. Report of General Porter. In Stewart CW, ed. *John Paul Jones: Commemoration at Annapolis,* April 24, 1906. Washington, DC: U.S. Government Printing Office, 1907:49–79.

17. Op. cit. Thomas, p. 15, 16.

18. Ibid., p. 17–21.

19. Ibid., p. 22.

20. Ibid., p. 30–33.

21. Ibid., p. 45.

22. Ibid., p. 195.

23. Ibid., p. 114.

24. Ibid., p. 150.

25. Ibid., p. 165.

26. Ibid., p. 212.

27. Ibid., pp. 219, 220, 231, 232.

28. Ibid., pp. 256, 257.

29. Ibid., p. 267.

30. Ibid., pp. 269–271.

31. Ibid., pp. 279–296.

32. Ibid., pp. 297–299.

33. Ibid., pp. 302, 303.

34. Capitan L. Report of Doctor Captain. In Stewart CW, ed. *John Paul Jones: Commemoration at Annapolis,* April 24, 1906. Washington, DC: U.S. Government Printing Office, 1907:81–85.

35. Cornil V. Report of Professor Cornil. In Stewart CW, ed. *John Paul Jones: Commemoration at Annapolis,* April 24, 1906. Washington, DC: U.S. Government Printing Office, 1907:93–94.

36. Weir MR, Bogle LL, Mackowiak PA. The death of John Paul Jones and resurrections as "father of the US Navy." *Am J Nephrol* 2010;31:90–94.

37. Gubler DJ. Dengue and dengue hemorrhagic fever. *Clin Microbiol Rev* 1998;11:480–496.

38. Berman SJ, Tsai CC, Holmes K, et al. Sporadic anicteric leptospirosis in South Vietnam. A study in 150 patients. *Ann Intern Med* 1973;79:167–173.

39. Mackowiak PA. *Post Mortem. Solving History's Great Medical Mysteries.* Philadelphia: ACP Press, 2007:224.

40. Kaehny WD, Ozawa T, Schwartz MT, et al. Acute nephritis and pulmonary alveolitis following pneumococcal pneumonia. *Arch Intern Med* 1978;138:806–809.

41. Forrest JW, John F, Mills LR, et al. Immune complex glomerulonephritis associated with *Klebsiella pneumoniae* infection. *Clin Nephrol* 1977;7:76–79.

42. Simou E, Kollios KD, Papadimitriou P, et al. Acute nephritis and respiratory tract infection caused by *Mycoplasma pneumoniae*: case report and review of the literature. *Pediatr Infect Dis J* 2003;22:1103–1107.

43. Ronco P, Verroust P, Morel-Maroger L. Viruses and glomerulonephritis. *Nephron* 1982;31:97–102.

44. Smith MC, Cooke JR, Zimmerman DM, et al. Asymptomatic glomerulonephritis after nonstreptococcal upper respiratory infections. *Ann Intern Med* 1979;91:697–702.

45. Op. cit. Mackowiak, pp. 173–202.

46. Epstein FH, Merrill JP. Chronic renal failure. In Thorn GW, Adams RD, Braunwald E, et al., eds. *Harrisons's Principles of Internal Medicine*, 8th ed. New York: McGraw-Hill Book Co., 1977:1435.

47. Lasky II. Autopsy of Admiral John Paul Jones 113 years postmortem. Historical and forensic aspects. *NY State J Med* 1982;June:1110–1115.

48. Neilson EG, Kelly CJ. Chronic interstitial nephritis. In Kelly WN, ed. *Textbook of Internal Medicine*, 2nd ed. Philadelphia: J. B. Lippincott Co., 1992:718–720.

49. Nriagu JO. Saturnine gout among Roman aristocrats. Did lead poisoning contribute to the fall of the empire? *N Engl J Med* 1983;308:660–663.

50. Józsa LG. Histologic diagnoses of tissues from two nineteenth century Habsburgs. *Paleopathol News L* 2008;141:12–18.

51. Donadio JV, Grande JP. IgA nephropathy. *N Engl J Med* 2002;347:738–748.

52. Suzuki H, Moldoveanu Z, Hall S, et al. IgA1-secreting cell lines from patients with IgA nephropathy produce aberrantly glycosylated IgA1. *J Clin Invest* 2008;118:629–639.

53. Buell AC. *Paul Jones: Founder of the American Navy*. New York: Charles Scribner and Sons, 1900.

54. Field E. Paul Jones, Founder of the American Navy, a history. *Am Historical Rev* 1901;April:589–590.

55. General Porter's Triumph. *New York Times,* April 16, 1905.

56. Theodore Roosevelt to Charles J. Bonaparte, August 1, 1905, reel 338, series 2, Theodore Roosevelt Papers, Library of Congress.

57. http://www.history.navy.mil/faqs/faq113–1.htm

6 *El Sordo*

WHAT A STRANGE artist this patient was. He was a nonconformist and a revolutionary, a singular genius who saw things invisible. And his method of painting was as eccentric as his talent. He "scooped his colour out of tubs, applied it with sponges, mops, rags, anything...he could lay his hands on. He trowelled and slapped his colours on like a bricklayer, giving characteristic touches with a stroke of his thumb. In this extemporary way he covered thirty feet or so of wall in a couple of days" (1).

He was one of the greatest portraitists of modern times. During his long career, he experimented continuously in new media and innovative artistic techniques as a draftsman, tapestry cartoonist, and engraver. He even mastered the novel technique of lithography in his twilight years. He is credited with an astonishing succession of decorative paintings, tapestry designs, portraits of Spanish nobles and kings, as well as images of humble workmen and farmers, sometimes injured or killed in the course of their toil. He produced works of art that attacked corruption, superstition, and vice in high and low places, during a maelstrom of confusion, misery, and repression such as Spain had never known before (2).

He produced over 1,800 works of art—some would say masterpieces—many of which have been lost. Such extraordinary productivity required nearly incomprehensible speed. It is said that he painted his wife's portrait, now hanging in the Prado, in an hour, and that he completed King Fernando's huge painting in just one or two sessions, that of the Infante Don Luis in a single morning. The frenetic pace of his work was all the more impressive because of its quality and charm.

No painter before or since executed a lifelike portrait so perfectly in so short a time. It is no wonder that he became the most sought-after portraitist in Madrid (2).

In the winter of 1792–93, he was attacked by a mysterious illness that nearly killed him. He survived but lost his hearing and for the next 35 years was "deaf as a stump" (3). The illness has generated endless speculation and nearly two dozen diagnoses because of who he was, and also because the character of his work changed so radically in its aftermath. Before the illness had destroyed his hearing, he painted gentle, colorful scenes of picnics and games and produced elegant tapestries and cartoons in the Rococo style. Afterward, many of his works were dark and nightmarish, with a merciless, often vengeful, view of the world (2, 4–7). Because the metamorphosis followed the illness, many have suspected that the illness was responsible for the change. However, his works were social documents in which he revolted against his country's fate no less than his own under the Spanish Bourbons, a newly invigorated Inquisition, and the ineffable indignities of a French occupation.

The patient was 46 when the illness struck. Until then, he had enjoyed robust health except for a brief, unspecified illness at age 32 (8), and 8 years after that, minor injuries suffered when a carriage he was taking for a test drive overturned (2, 5). According to letters and other contemporary documents, the illness that destroyed his hearing and nearly killed him lasted several months. For 2 months he was too ill to leave his bed. Whether the illness came on gradually or all of a sudden or if it involved fever is not known. What is known is that it caused loud buzzing and roaring in his ears, and then mounting deafness. In the initial phase of the illness, he had difficulty maintaining his balance and for a long time could not go up or down stairs without feeling in danger of falling (4). He was nauseated, complained of abdominal pain (5, 6), and had no appetite. During the worst of the illness, he fainted intermittently and had difficulty seeing. He was also confused, hallucinated repeatedly, and had temporary bouts of partial paralysis (2, 7). Eventually he recovered his faculties, including his eyesight. However, never again did he hear a sound.

Neither the patient nor any of the physicians he might have consulted had the knowledge to diagnose, much less cure, his disorder. If he was seen by a doctor, we have no record of such and, hence, are handicapped greatly in efforts to give his illness a name. In any case, the patient had a low regard for the profession, portraying physicians in his works as fraudulent, incompetent, rapacious asses. He was neither alone nor unjustified in this regard. Indeed, Voltaire, a contemporary of his, advised that: "Men must have religion and not believe in priests, just as men must have a diet and not believe in physicians." The public's disdain for the profession was no less biting. They derided physicians as *matassanos* ("killers of the healthy") and surgeons as *sangradores*, "blood-letters" (9). The deplorable absence of medical competence in Spain of the patient's day was the legacy of restrictions on scientific thought imposed by the Church and enforced by the Inquisition, in addition to the Church's insistence that physical explanations of illness were of necessity subordinate to metaphysical explanations (7). The great wave of enlightenment that was the Renaissance had yet to wash away the ignorance, confusion, and superstition that had stifled innovative thought in Spain since the reign of Isabel and Fernando (10).

The patient was born on March 30, 1746, in Zaragoza, the capital of the province of Aragón, halfway between Madrid and the French border. His father, José, was a master gilder. His mother, Gracia Lucientes, was the daughter of an hidalgo (*hijo de algo*—"the son of someone"). They had six children, four sons and two daughters. The patient was the fourth child (11, 12). Little is known of his early education other than that he attended the Escuela Pías de San Antón, a church school that offered free education to gifted children of the poor. Many years later he produced one of the most piercing and beautiful images of old age in a commemorative altarpiece of the school's founder, San José de Calasanz, raising himself from his deathbed to receive Holy Communion. One of the patient's fellow pupils, Martín Zapater, became a close, lifelong friend. They exchanged some 131 letters between 1755 and 1801, which contain most of what we know of the patient's medical history (13).

With regard to the patient's education as an artist, we know a bit more. At age 13 he was apprenticed to José Luzán, a local painter who had trained under Guiseppe Mastroleo in Naples. Luzán taught him the rudiments of design and made him copy the best prints he owned. After 4 years with Luzán, the patient decided to travel to Italy to see, to study, and to absorb the high reaches of Italian art. When he arrived, the titans of the past were all dead; Bellini, Titian, Michelangelo, Raphael, Correggio, and all the rest lived on only in their works (14). Little is known of the patient's Italian sojourn or how it influenced his art, if at all. Much later he would allow only that "He had no other master than his own observation of famous paintings and painters in Rome and Spain, from which he drew greatest profit" (2).

The patient was by nature a *majo*, a tough guy of the city, who as a youth liked to wear the tight breeches, stockings, and sash with the embroidered "suit of lights" of a bullfighter (15) (Fig. 6.1). The attire complemented his compact, sturdy frame of medium height. This image resulted in not a few myths promulgated by early biographers. Among them were ones claiming that as a youth he was the ringleader of a gang of delinquents, whose escapades led to his awaking one morning with a knife in his back; that he left Madrid for Italy with a troupe of bullfighters to escape the

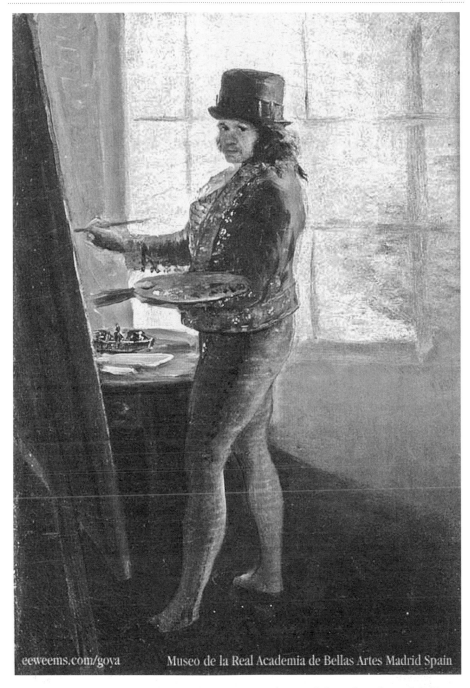

FIGURE 6.1 The patient as a young man. Self-portrait. (Museo de la Real Academia de Bellas Artes de San Fernando, Madrid)

Inquisition; that he had to flee Rome on account of more wild behavior—trying to abduct a young nun with whom he had become infatuated from her convent (16). There is no evidence to support any of these romantic stories (17).

He married Josepha Bayeu, the sister of a fellow painter, when he was 28. Although there have been rumors that he was not always faithful, the marriage lasted without incident or scandal for 39 years. Josepha had over a score of pregnancies, from which only six children were brought to term. Just one son, Javier, born in 1784, survived infancy (18).

The patient's rise to greatness as an artist, social critic, and philosopher is all the more remarkable because Spain had for so long cultivated and preserved unsullied intellectual mediocrity on behalf of the Church and through the vigilance of the Inquisition. During the patient's day, there was no strong, inventive bourgeoisie to challenge church dogma. There was only an excess of priests and aristocrats determined to keep the populace illiterate, disenfranchised, and stupefied with prayer and patriotism. The enlightened ideas of the Age of Reason, which convulsed and remade European thought during the 18th century, "stopped at the Pyrenees and [were] heard below them only as dull echoes, faint chirpings, ill-understood threats to the order of things" (19). This deaf patient was one of the few who heard them. And when the "little war" with Napoleon pillaged, eviscerated, and bankrupted Spain, he recorded and rebelled against the atrocities of both sides in works that resonate no less today than they did then.

In 1819, when the patient was 73, he was again seriously ill. Little is known of the nature of the illness other than that the physician who cared for him, Dr. Eugenio García Arrieta, was a yellow fever expert (20). The patient commemorated the illness and his physician in an *ex voto* portrait thanking Arrieta for having saved his life (Fig. 6.2). As with many of the patient's works, this one is allegorical and subject to all manner of interpretations (9, 21).

The patient's final years were unsettled by the ascension of Fernando VII to the Spanish throne following Napoleon's defeat. Fernando was a reactionary ruler who supported slavery, judicial torture, imprisonment without trial, and strict censorship. He had no use for even the most elementary human rights, regarding them as a threat to his absolute power (22). The patient feared that he too would fall victim to Fernando's tyranny and on September 17, 1823, deeded his house, *Quinta del Sordo*, "the deaf man's house", to his grandson, Mariano, as he prepared to quit Madrid forever (23). He was old, arthritic, tired, and nearly blind. However, he was optimistic despite his infirmities. Already master nonpareil of etching, he embarked upon the conquest of a new technique, lithography (24).

He found his way to Bordeaux, where he bought a comfortable house of brick and adobe on 22 acres of arable land. He brought a housekeeper with him from Madrid

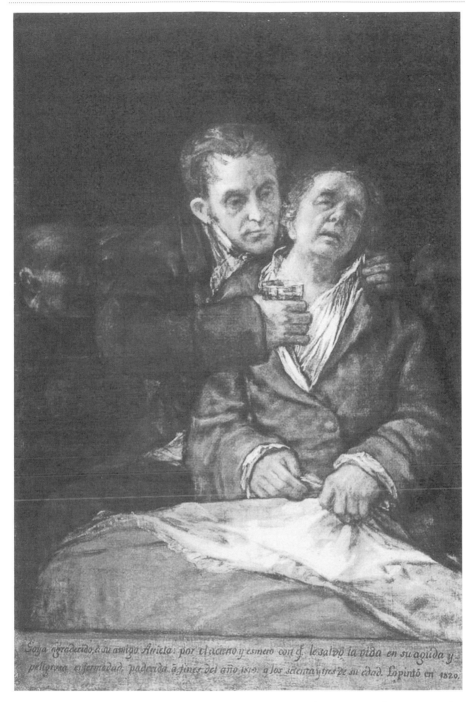

FIGURE 6.2 Self-portrait of the patient with Dr. Arrieta, 1820. (The Minneapolis Institute of the Arts)

named Leocadia Zorilla de Weis, "about whom not much is known but quite a lot has been assumed." Leocadia was attractive and many years younger than he, and when she gave birth to a daughter, Rosaria, in October 1814, 2 years after the death of Josepha, it was assumed that the patient was the child's father (25).

The patient's health was deteriorating (26). In 1825 he complained of problems urinating. His doctors diagnosed paralysis of the bladder. An enormous tumor had grown on one of his legs. He began taking valerian, a sedative derived from the herb of the same name, which made him feel stronger. However, the improvement was an illusion. On April 2, 1828, he was found unconscious on the floor of his studio, paintbrush in hand (27). He lingered in a coma for 2 weeks, speechless and unresponsive, his right side paralyzed. Finally, on April 16, Francisco José de Goya y Lucientes (Fig. 6.3) died.

The next day, after a Mass was said for the repose of his soul, Goya was interred in the cemetery of the Chartreuse in Bordeaux. In 1901, when the Spanish government asked for the remains of one of her greatest sons to be returned, they were transferred to Madrid. In 1929, the government decided to rebury Goya

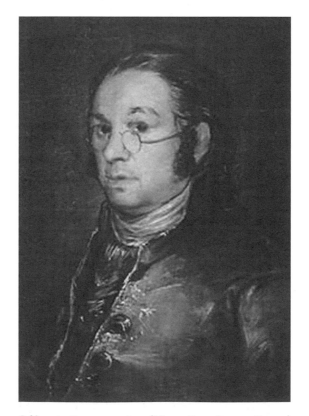

FIGURE 6.3   Goya. Self-portrait, c. 1797–1800. (Musee Goya Castres, France)

under the floor of Santa María de la Florida, which he had so beautifully decorated. When the body was exhumed this time, the skull was missing and has yet to be found (26).

The cause of Goya's death is no mystery. He was 82 years old when he died. His health had been declining steadily for some time due to the ravages of old age on his arteries, eyes, bladder, joints, and bones. Death finally arrived in the form of a massive cerebral infarction. What is a mystery, one for which an answer has yet to be found, is the name (the diagnosis) of the disorder that robbed him of his hearing when he was 46 and what effect it had on his work.

Most early biographers thought syphilis, specifically meningovascular syphilis (syphilis of the brain and its surrounding membranes), was the illness responsible for Goya's deafness (16). They argued that the high prevalence of the infection in Europe at the time (an estimated 10% of the population is thought to have been infected (28)) and the (alleged) wild escapades of the artist's youth placed him, as the statisticians might put it, "at considerable risk" of the venereal infection. Moreover, the clinical constellation of visual difficulties, deafness, and temporary paralysis, combined with abnormal behavior, was deemed highly suggestive of syphilis involving the small arteries of the brain and spinal cord. Goya's lifelong friend and confidant, Martín Zapater, fanned the flame of such speculation by stating that the illness was the result of Goya's "own lack of reflection" (2). Then there was the matter of Josepha's obstetrical difficulties. Allegedly, she had some 20 pregnancies, from which only one child survived. Some believe that Goya's depiction of Saturn gorging himself on one of his progeny (Fig. 6.4) was inspired by the artist's guilt and self-loathing for having infected Josepha with syphilis and thereby having been responsible for the death of so many of his children (9).

Before the advent of penicillin, congenital syphilis did devour many children in utero, as well as in infancy. However, syphilis was but one of many causes of such deaths. Moreover, today biographers are no longer sure of the number of Josepha's pregnancies and suspect that she might have had far fewer than earlier reported (2). Perhaps most important, meningovascular syphilis is a progressive disorder. It is inconceivable that it could have assaulted Goya, rapidly destroyed his hearing, nearly killed him, and then receded so completely for another 38 years that the artist was able not just to live and to work, but to produce some of his greatest art.

In Goya's day, artists ground their own pigments, which they mixed with various solvents to produce paints. Lead white, which contained copious amounts of lead, was one of Goya's principal pigments. He primed his canvasses with successive layers of it combined with linseed oil to produce a smooth painting surface. His portrait of the Marquesa de Pontejos and his famous *Burial of the Sardine* are

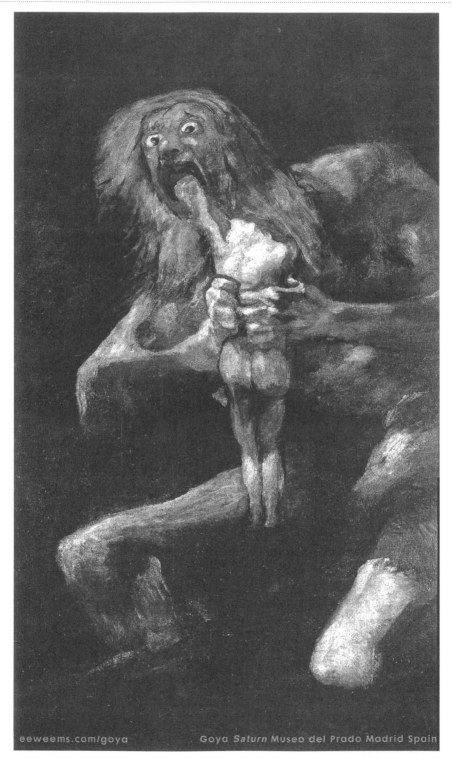

FIGURE 6.4 Goya, *Saturno devorando a suhijo* (Saturn Devouring His Son), 1820–24. Oil transferred to canvas from mural. (Museo Nacional del Prado, Madrid)

examples in which such priming was used liberally. Both were painted prior to his 1792–93 illness. It has been theorized that grinding the huge amount of lead contained in the white lead he used as an undercoat placed Goya at considerable risk of lead intoxication due to repeated inhalation and ingestion of the aerosolized metal. He would have been especially prone to such intoxication because the tremendous speed with which he worked potentially increased his exposure via inhalation to all manner of noxious substances used to produce his paints. This seems to have been an occupational hazard of artists of that era, as reflected by the following observation by Ramazzini in 1713: "I have observed that nearly all the painters whom I know, both in this or other cities, are sickly... for their liability to disease [because of] the materials of colors that they handle and smell constantly" (2).

Beethoven also lost his hearing, though gradually, and there are those who believe that his deafness, like Goya's, was due to lead intoxication (plumbism) (29). Colic is one of plumbism's most prominent symptoms, manifesting as abdominal pain, cramps, nausea, and loss of appetite, which were features of Goya's 1792–93 illness. Lead is also toxic to nerves, impairing their ability to conduct the electrical impulses that stimulate muscles to contract. Weakness and sometimes paralysis are the usual result. Although the acoustic nerves can be injured, they are normally spared. For this reason, lead intoxication is an unlikely cause of Goya's deafness. In addition, there is no evidence that Goya used less lead carbonate-based pigment in the years after his illness than before (9), making it difficult to incriminate lead as the cause of either his deafness or the other serious but transient symptoms with which he suffered so intensely during the illness.

Two immunological disorders of unknown etiology have also been proposed as the cause of Goya's deafness—the Vogt-Koyanagi-Harada (V-K-H) syndrome and Cogan's syndrome. Both have features similar to those of Goya's 1792–93 illness. Terence Cawthorne, an English ophthalmologist, first proposed the V-K-H syndrome as Goya's diagnosis in 1961 (16). The syndrome is a systemic disorder in which the immune system turns against the host (i.e., it is an "autoimmune" disorder). Melanocytes (pigment-producing cells) are the principal target of the renegade inflammatory cells responsible for the disorder. The skin, hair, eye (retina), nervous system, and ear all contain melanocytes, the destruction of which leads to vitiligo (nonpigmented patches of white skin), poliosis (patches of white hair in the scalp, brows, or lashes), and inflammation of the eyes, meninges, and inner ear. The disorder is extremely rare. Women are affected more often than men. Headache, increased sensitivity to touch, vertigo, nausea, neck stiffness, vomiting, and low-grade fever are early symptoms. Patients usually seek medical attention because of eye complaints, such as loss of vision, eye pain, and/or light intolerance (photophobia). Deafness and dizziness are less prominent (30–32).

After weeks to months, most patients develop the cutaneous abnormalities listed above, which Goya apparently did not.

Cogan's syndrome, another multisystem disorder of unknown origin (also presumed to be an autoimmune disease), has even more features similar to those of Goya's illness (33, 34). Vestibulo-auditory dysfunction and nonsyphilitic interstitial keratitis (inflammation of the wall of the eye) are its principal abnormalities. The vestibulo-auditory dysfunction begins abruptly with attacks of vertigo, ataxia (loss of balance), tinnitus (ringing/buzzing in the ears), nausea, vomiting, and sudden hearing loss. Eye problems sometimes develop simultaneously, but in others as long as 1 to 2 years later. Occasionally, the disorder attacks blood vessels throughout the body, causing them to become inflamed and producing systemic symptoms such as fever, headache, seizures, hallucinations, psychosis, and abdominal pain. Although the disorder can develop at any age, the median age at onset is 25. Spontaneous resolution of Cogan's syndrome having manifestations as severe as those of Goya's illness after only a few months, with no apparent recurrence during the next 38 years, would be highly unusual.

Common things are common, and when a bizarre illness such as Goya's is finally diagnosed, it is generally a common disorder presenting in an uncommon way rather than a rare disorder presenting in typical fashion. The best example of this principle is exhibited by patients with "fevers of unknown origin"—fevers defying diagnosis in spite of intensive investigation. In virtually every published series of such cases, diagnoses, when finally made, are predominantly atypical cases of common disorders rather than typical cases of rare disorders (35). Goya's illness, I believe, is best explained by an atypical case of a common infection.

Goya was an avid hunter (8) and, hence, potentially was exposed to ticks carrying *Borrelia burgdorferi*, the agent responsible for Lyme disease. Lyme disease is the most common arthropod-borne disease in both Europe and the United States. If untreated, approximately 15 percent of patients develop neurological abnormalities, such as meningitis, encephalitis, and inflammation of the cranial nerves. The auditory nerve, one of the cranial nerves, can be attacked, but less often than the facial nerve, another cranial nerve (36). Thus, facial paralysis, sometimes bilateral, is more common than vestibulo-auditory dysfunction. The infection rarely if ever causes bilateral deafness (Wormser, G., personal communication).

Except for his abdominal pain, all of Goya's symptoms during his 1792–93 illness point to a disorder of the brain, specifically an acute infection of the brain—an encephalitis. His fainting spells, transient paralysis, visual difficulties, and intermittent confusion and hallucinations are all typical of encephalitis. His vestibulo-auditory problems (tinnitus, vertigo, and deafness) were likely due to collateral damage to the inner ear caused by the encephalitis rather than destruction of auditory centers within the brain itself. Only an infection of the brain, an encephalitis, is likely to produce symptoms of the sort experienced by Goya, almost kill the patient while destroying completely his hearing, and then subside without treatment. An untreated bacterial encephalitis would not have done so, since nearly all such untreated cases are fatal. Goya's disorder was almost certainly a viral encephalitis, one that eventually resolved without treatment because his immune system overcame it before it killed him.

A host of viruses are responsible for human cases of encephalitis (37). Many, such as the West Nile virus responsible for the recent epidemic in the United States, are transmitted by mosquitoes. Encephalitis caused by such viruses typically occurs during the warm months of the year, when mosquitoes are most active. Goya's illness developed in late December or early January and hence is unlikely to have been due to an arbovirus, one of the viruses transmitted by mosquitoes.

Measles (38, 39) and mumps (40–42) are two viral infections prevalent during the winter months. Both were exceedingly common prior to the 1960s, when vaccines effective against them were introduced. Both viruses cause encephalitis in humans. Although encephalitis is a rare complication of these infections, adults are more likely to develop the complication than children. Both types of encephalitis can cause deafness—the former by facilitating bacterial invasion of the middle ear and the latter by a direct attack on the vestibulo-auditory nerves (Fig. 6.5). Mumps occasionally also attacks the pancreas, which could explain the nausea and abdominal pain Goya experienced during his 1792–93 illness. Because mumps is less contagious than measles, Goya would have been more likely to have escaped that infection than measles until the age of 46, when finally infected by his son, Javier, who was then 7 years old.

Thus, of all the disorders that might explain Goya's deafness, none offers a better fit with the character and the course of his illness than mumps encephalitis. Although encephalitis is a rare complication of mumps, the infection itself was extremely common before the advent of modern immunization, when it was the most common cause of viral encephalitis in temperate regions of the world. Before the introduction of an effective vaccine, mumps was also one of the leading causes of deafness in children and young adults (42). Mumps encephalitis can be severe in adults, occasionally even fatal. Clinically it is manifested by confusion, convulsions, partial paralysis, impaired speech (aphasia), and involuntary movements. In one case series, permanent deafness developed as a complication of mumps encephalitis in 9 percent of the patients surveyed (41). Eye abnormalities are not a feature of mumps in general or mumps encephalitis in particular. Therefore, if Goya's "spells of semi-blindness" were due to mumps encephalitis, likely they

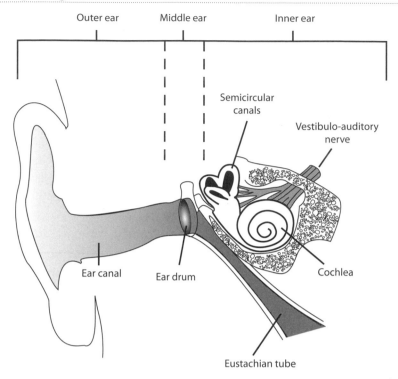

Outer ear   Middle ear   Inner ear

Semicircular
canals

Vestibulo-auditory
nerve

Ear canal   Ear drum   Cochlea

Eustachian tube

FIGURE 6.5 Drawing of the inner ear showing the location of the vestibulo-auditory (balance-hearing) nerve in relation to the semicircular canal (the sensory organ responsible for maintaining balance or equilibrium) and the cochlea (the principal hearing organ).

would have been the result of inflammation of the area of the brain responsible for processing visual signals, the occipital lobe, rather than a problem with the eyes themselves.

The effect of Goya's illness and his deafness on his work has long been argued. One obvious effect was that his deafness forced him to resign from teaching at the Royal Academy in Madrid. He found that he had "lost all hope of giving any assistance, since [he] was unable to hear anything that the pupils said...and this led to general amusement among the boys and disruption of the class" (7). The character of his work also changed radically after his illness. When his hearing was gone, his mind and his work turned to disaster and mayhem (43). He became an alcolophile, a lover of ugliness, (44), whose nearly every work carried the stamp of scorn (45). And yet, it has been speculated that only then did he achieve full mastery of the face in his portraits (46). Once he had lost his hearing, his skills as a portraitist deepened, possibly because deafness made him more aware of gesture, physical expression, and all the minute particulars of how faces and bodies reveal themselves.

This transformation followed Goya's illness, but was it caused by his illness? Did his deafness cause him to rebel against his fate through his art and produce the morbid images that populated later works, or were other traumas of his private life responsible—his wife's miscarriages, his country's agony under the yoke of a corrupt administration, and later the ravages of the Peninsular War? The answers to these questions can never be known for certain. What is certain is that this was an artist who perceived more than his fellows and recorded more than he saw (47). His works are a source of eternal wonder and delight that speak to the sense of mystery surrounding our lives no less forcefully today than when he was alive, as they do to our sense of beauty and pity and pain (48).

References

1. Gautier T. *Voyage en Espagne* (Travels in Spain), 1843.

2. Niederland WG. Goya's illness. A case of lead encephalopathy? *NY State J Med* 1972;72:413–418.

3. Connell ES. *Francisco Goya. Life and Times.* New York: Counterpoint, 2004:201.

4. Hughes R. *Goya.* New York: Alfred A. Knopf, 2006:127–128.

5. Ravin JG, Ravin TB. What ailed Goya? *Surv Ophthalmol* 1999;44:263–270.

6. Park MP, Park RHR. The fine art of patient–doctor relationship. *Br Med J* 2004;329:1475–1480.

7. Mathiasen H. Emphatic art: Goya and Dr. Arrieta. *Am J Med* 2008;121:355–356.

8. Op. cit. Hughes, p. 116.

9. Casey LL. Goya: "in sickness and in health." *Int J Surg* 2006;4:66–72.

10. Op. cit. Connell, p. 64.

11. Ibid., p. 6.

12. Op. cit. Hughes, p. 27.

13. Ibid., p. 32.

14. Ibid., pp. 33–36.

15. Ibid., p. 80–81.

16. Cawthorne T. Goya's illness. *Proc Roy Soc Med* 1962;55:213–217.

17. Op. cit. Hughes, p. 37.

18. Ibid., p. 38.

19. Ibid., p. 68.

20. Ibid., p. 373.

21. Claman HN. Portraits: Goya and his physician, Dr. Arrieta. *The Pharos* 2008 (Winter):8–11.

22. Op. cit. Hughes, pp. 320–324.

23. Ibid., p. 388.

24. Ibid., pp. 390–391.

25. Ibid., pp. 372–373.

26. Ibid., pp. 400–402.

27. Op. cit. Connell, pp. 232–233.

28. Mackowiak PA. *Post Mortem. Solving History's Great Medical Mysteries.* Philadelphia ACP Press, 2007:224.

29. Ibid., pp. 215–217.

30. Snyder DA, Tessler HH. Vogt-Koyanagi-Harada syndrome. *Am J Ophthalmol* 1980;90:69–75.

31. Bykhovskaya I, Thorne JE, Kempen JH, et al. Vogt-Koyanagi-Harada disease: clinical outcomes. *Am J Ophthalmol* 2005;140:674–678.

32. Sil A, Chatrath P, Gatland DJ. Deafness in Vogt-Koyanagi-Harada syndrome. *J Laryngol* 2006;120:416–418.

33. Vollersten RS, McDonald TJ, Younge BR, et al. Cogan's syndrome: 18 cases and a review of the literature. *Mayo Clinic Proc* 1986;61:344–361.

34. St. Clair EW, McCallum RM. Cogan's syndrome. In Hochberg MC, Silman AJ. Smolen JS, et al., eds. *Rheumatology*, 5th ed. Philadelphia: Mosby Elsevier, 2011:1625–1634.

35. Mackowiak PA, Durack DT. Fever of unknown origin. In Mandell GL, Bennett JE, Dolin R, eds. *Principles and Practice of Infectious Diseases*, 7th ed. Philadelphia: Churchill Livingstone Elsevier, 2010:779–781.

36. Steere AC. *Borrelia burgdorferi* (Lyme disease, Lyme borreliosis). In Mandell GL, Bennett JE, Dolin R, eds. *Principles and Practice of Infectious Diseases*, 7th ed. Philadelphia: Churchill Livingstone Elsevier, 2010:3071–3081.

37. Whitley RJ. Viral encephalitis. *N Engl J Med* 1990;323:242–250.

38. Gershon AA. Measles virus (rubeola). In Mandell GL, Bennett JE, Dolin R, eds. *Principles and Practice of Infectious Diseases*, 7th ed. Philadelphia: Churchill Livingstone Elsevier, 2010:2229–2236.

39. MMR Disease Information—NVIC (Measles). Available online at www.nvic.org/vaccines-and-Diseases/MMR.aspx (accessed May 1, 2012).

40. Litman N, Baum SG. Mumps virus. In Mandell GL, Bennett JE, Dolin R, eds. *Principles and Practice of Infectious Diseases*, 7th ed. Philadelphia: Churchill Livingstone Elsevier, 2010:2201–2206.

41. Association for the Study of Infectious Disease. A retrospective survey of the complications of mumps. *J Roy Coll Gen Practitioners* 1974;24:552–556.

42. MUMPS, Mumps virus, mumps infection. Available online at http://virology-online.com/viruses/MUMPS.htm (accessed May 1, 2012).

43. Op. cit. Hughes, p. 135.

44. Op. cit. Connell, p. 123.

45. Ibid., p. 129.

46. Op. cit. Hughes, p. 165.

47. Craig EG. *On the Art of the Theatre*. 1911.

48. Conrad J. *The Nigger of the `Narcissus'* (preface). 1897.

Am I so ill that I need to give my last testament and make my confession?...How will I get out of this labyrinth?

The patient on his deathbed to Dr. Révérend, December 1830

7 A Medical Labyrinth

NORTH AMERICANS KNOW this patient's name but very little else about him, and yet none of the heroes of South America ranks higher in accomplishments as a soldier and statesman or was more admired in his day by Americans and Europeans for his struggle to institute liberty where tyranny had reigned (1, 2). His exploits, more than those of anyone, were responsible for Spain's loss of its trans-Atlantic colonies. According to Hiram Bingham of *The Geographical Journal* (3): "His passage of the Andes was mightier than Hannibal's passage of the Alps; his marches were longer than those of Genghis Khan and Tamerlane; his audacity in risking odds equaled Marlborough's, while his patience under reverse, his skills in heading dispirited, half-mutinous armies and his never failing ingenuity as a strategist entitled him to the praises, somewhat grudgingly bestowed by Wellington, of being an extraordinary commander."

Bingham's hyperbole aside, this patient's feats of endurance and his accomplishments were nothing short of astonishing. He founded three republics and was the primary magistrate of three countries (1), two of which now bear his name. He was revered by the likes of Lafayette, Lord Byron, and George Washington's family (4, 5). For a time while he lived, he was idealized and mythologized until the brilliance of his persona exceeded that of even his extraordinary legacy. However, when he had run the race that fate allotted, he died "in a modest countryside house, poor, persecuted and accompanied by only a few friends and faithful servants" (1).

Prior to the patient's emergence as revolutionary leader, apart from Brazil and the three Guyanas, the continent of South America was ruled by Spain for nearly

300 years. Together with José San Martin, the national hero of Argentina, he wrested from Spanish domination a New World empire five times as vast as that of all of Europe (6). His conquests, which began in 1811, involved some 100 battles and covered nearly 80,000 miles of forced marches (7). In 1819, he liberated New Granada (present-day Colombia and Panama) as victor in the battle of Boyacá; in 1821, Venezuela (battle of Carabobo); in 1822, Ecuador (battle of Pinchincha); in 1824, Perú (battles of Junín and Ayacucho); and in 1825, Bolivia (as victor in the battle of Tumusla, his last battle), freeing the bulk of Spain's American empire (8). Throughout these campaigns, he fought in the front lines without receiving a scratch, moving "through enemy fire with such thoughtless serenity that his officers accepted the easy explanation that he believed himself invulnerable" (9).

He began life in Caracas on July 24, 1783. His parents were Spanish-Americans of Basque descent (10). Both reputedly died of tuberculosis (11)—his father at age 56, when the patient was 2 years old, and his mother at age 33, when he was 9. However, his father was a notorious womanizer (12), and some have speculated that paralytic syphilis killed him, and that congenital syphilis was responsible for the death of a daughter, the patient's sister, shortly after birth (12). There were three other siblings, an older brother and two older sisters. None is known to have developed either syphilis or tuberculosis. His sisters died at ages 65 and 68 of unknown cause (12), and his brother was lost at sea at age 30 while returning from the United States with a shipment of arms and ammunition meant for the patient's First Republic (13).

The patient married when he was 18, only to lose his young bride 8 months later to "malignant fever" (probably yellow fever) (14). He never remarried but had numerous subsequent affairs with mistresses and prostitutes, none of which is known to have produced an offspring (15). Although many of his hussars and grenadiers contracted the "fiery seed" of venereal disease (16), he seems never to have been touched by such infections.

During his prime, the patient was slightly below medium height (5'6"), slim, and graceful. He ate frugally, avoided spirits and tobacco (17), and enjoyed reasonably good health throughout most of his life in spite of the privations and stresses of commanding an army at war for 20 years in some of South America's most inhospitable terrain. Whereas his complexion was very white as a youth, by age 44 it had become dark and rough (18). An unsubstantiated report states that "His genital organs [were] small, the testes hard and the cords short" (19).

When the patient was 29 and campaigning in the Magdalena River basin in north-central Colombia, he had an attack of *fiebre aguda* (acute fever) and furunculosis (a pustular skin eruption) of unknown etiology, from which he recovered (20). Throughout the ensuing decade, he had repeated bouts of fever, during at least some of which he at first "looked flushed and then pale and shivering with cold…and then lost consciousness" (21). These were treated in some instances with quinine and in others with arsenic. On one occasion, the latter treatment is reported to have induced a severe attack of "dysentery" (22). Although he was chronically constipated and also suffered with recurrent "colic," "rheumatism," and painful hemorrhoids (23), he was reasonably fit until age 40, when he developed a high fever and collapsed, possibly as a result of heat stroke (24). For 7 days he hovered near death in a small village north of Lima, and for 2 months he was so weak and emaciated that he was hardly recognizable. Nevertheless, within 4 months, he had recovered sufficiently to lead his army to Pasco in central Perú, elevation 13,973 feet, over some of the most mountainous country in the world (3).

"[The patient's] temperament was a peculiar mixture of resolution and indecision, liberalism and authoritarianism, generosity and cruelty, and narcissistic vainglory" (25). During his myriad illnesses, he "was indifferent to his condition and refused to be looked after by a physician" (1). It was claimed that he felt an unconquerable repugnance for cures and believed that his bad temper, his *atrabilis*, was the principal cause of his ills (26). When at last he did enlist medical help, the sepulcher was already open and only a miracle could have saved him from descending therein (1).

Unfortunately for this patient, medicine did not yet have the capacity to perform miracles. It had no well-defined concept of infection or immunity, no vaccines, and, except for quinine, no effective treatments for any of the infections that attacked the patient throughout his years of campaigning. Hippocratic doctrine, with its humoral theory and treatments (see Chapter 2 in *Post Mortem. Solving History's Great Medical Mysteries* (27)), had not yet released its grip on medical thought. Not until half a century later, as a result of the work of Koch, Davaine, Pasteur, and the like, was it realized how varied diseases actually were with regard to the legions of different microbes responsible for them. Because the critical importance of clean water and basic sanitation and hygiene for the prevention for epidemic infections remained largely unknown in the patient's time, war-borne microbes killed many more soldiers than battle wounds and decided the outcome of more campaigns than generals (28).

Exactly when this general's final illness began is uncertain. Although some believe the first symptoms of the pulmonary disorder that carried him off appeared at age 35 (20), others claim that except for the sicknesses described above, he was physically fit until age 45, when his health began to crumble (29). By then combat had ceased for want of royalist combatants, and he had come to realize that reform was vastly more difficult than revolution. His magnificent obsession of creating a *Gran Colombia*—a single nation, free and united from Mexico to Cape Horn—proved to be a roost of false dreams (30). He had become all-powerful, only to learn that by becoming so he needed to fear everything and everyone.

When he left Bogotá for Cartagena and exile in early 1830, the streets were mobbed with people rejoicing at his departure and burning his portraits (31). He was already so ill and wasted, and in such low spirits, that he could barely walk across the room. Although he longed for a little sherry and a glass of beer, or his favorite vegetables, keeping food down was difficult. He coughed constantly and struggled for breath.

He survived, though barely, another 10 months before arriving in Santa Marta on the evening of December 1, 1830, where he was met by a U.S. Navy surgeon, George MacNight, and a French doctor, Alexandre Prospère Révérend. Both agreed that the seat of his illness was his lungs (32). Révérend had trained in Paris under two of the most eminent clinicians of that era, Dupuytren and Laennec (the inventor of the stethoscope). He attended the patient daily during his final fortnight and on each occasion made detailed records of his findings, opinion, and treatments (1).

When first seen by Révérend, the patient was apathetic, emaciated, weak, and so dyspneic that he could no longer walk. He looked like a corpse that had escaped from the grave, with sharp pointed knees, thin calves, and a hollow weak voice. He complained of "pain in the base of [his] liver." His countenance was yellow. He coughed constantly, producing copious green sputum. He also hiccoughed a great deal. Interestingly, his sense of smell was unusually keen. This was apparent when one of his devoted friends, General J. M. Sardá, came for a farewell visit shortly before the patient died. Having saluted the patient, the general took a seat near his former commander. The patient said: "Please move your chair away a little." Sardá obliged. "A little more." Sardá complied. "Still more," repeated the patient. While altering his position further, Sardá said, "Allow me to say, your Excellency, that I have not realized that I was so dirty." "It's not that," said the patient. "It's that you smell of the devil." "How do you mean 'of the devil'?" asked Sardá. "That is to say, of your pipe," replied the patient. Whether the patient's sense of smell had always been so keen, or it had increased in acuity during his illness, is uncertain (1).

Over the ensuing 16 days, the patient continued coughing and was intermittently febrile, with hot head and cold extremities. His pulse was thready. Initially he was brighter during the day than at night, but slept little and gradually drifted into delirium. There were also episodes of indigestion and vomiting, sternal pain and then pain in both the right and left flanks, a sore tongue, which was dry, rough, and colored along its edges, and urinary incontinence (1).

Throughout this phase of the illness, the General received a panoply of drugs, potions, poultices, and maneuvers. He was given "pectoral remedies" mixed with narcotics and expectorants together with small doses of quinine sulfate to tone up his stomach. He was fed sago cakes, chicken, and soup. Turpentine poultices were applied to his chest along with an anodyne ointment to relieve his pain. A sedative was administered to suppress his cough and to calm him. He was given foot baths and had his hands immersed in tepid water to restore "the balance of the humors." Purgatives and enemas were administered in an unsuccessful attempt to relieve his chronic constipation. These were accompanied by blistering plasters derived from Cantharides beetles, gum Arabic, antispasmodics, cold compresses, leg rubs, mustard plasters, linseed water for his burning urine, and Gondret's pomade (a concoction of beef marrow and ammonia) (1).

When the end was near, the patient's breathing became a death rattle, his visage a *facies Hippocratica*, the face of a dead man. The small amount of urine he produced was bloody. In the early morning of December 17, 1830, "the gates of heaven groaned on their hinges" (33) to admit Simón José Antonio de la Santísima Trinidad Bolívar y Palacios (Fig. 7.1).

He was only 47, too soon bereft of youth and manly vigor and weighing barely 50 pounds. Révérend, who performed an autopsy later that day, diagnosed "tuberculous consumption" based on the following findings (1):

1. *Appearance of the body.*
   Cadaver in state of two thirds of decay; universal discolouration; swelling in the sacral region; musculature very little discoloured—normal consistency.
2. *Head.*
   The arachnoid vessels in the posterior half [were] slightly injected; the irregularities and convolutions of the cerebrum [were] covered by a brownish material with the consistency and transparency of gelatin; [there was] a little semi-red serous material beneath the dura mater; the rest of the cerebrum and cerebellum did not demonstrate any pathological abnormality.
3. *Chest.*
   Posteriorly and superiorly on both sides the pleurae were adherent as the result of semi-membranous material; there was hardening of the superior two thirds of each lung. The right, which was almost completely disorganised, looked like a fountain [sic] the colour of wine dregs studded with tubercles of different sizes—not very soft. The left lung although less disorganised showed the same tuberculous affection. Dividing this with a scalpel I found an irregular, angular, calcareous concretion about the size of a hazelnut. On opening the rest of the lungs with the instrument, I spilled some brown serous material which as a result of the pressure was rather frothy. The heart did not demonstrate anything particular although it was bathed in a liquid of a light green colour which was contained within the pericardium.

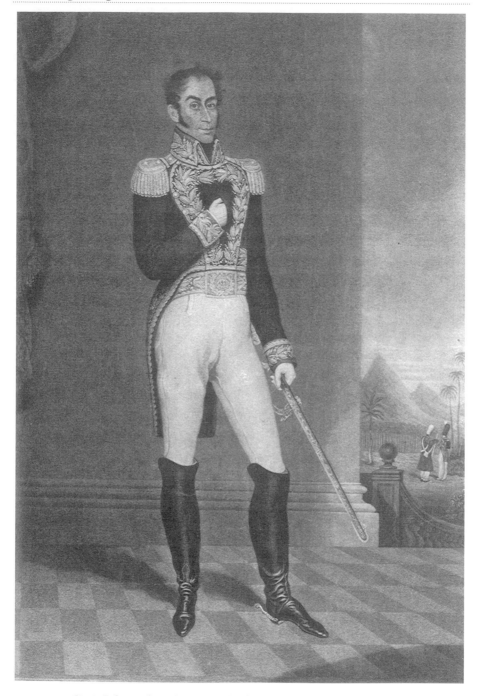

FIGURE 7.1 *Simón Bolívar, Libertador de Colombia*, by José Gil de Castro, Lima, 1827. Portrait currently resides in the John Carter Brown Library at Brown University.

4. *Abdomen.*

The stomach [was] dilated by a yellowish fluid with which its walls were heavily impregnated but nonetheless it did not show any lesions or inflammation. The intestines [were] attenuated and showed slight evidence of tympanites. The bladder [was] completely empty; it was collapsed and lying low in the pelvis; it did not exhibit any pathological signs. The liver [was] of a considerable size and was a little excoriated on its convex surface. The gall bladder [was] much extended. The mesenteric glands [were] obstructed. The spleen and kidneys were healthy. In general the visceral organs did not suffer from any serious lesions.

How well do these facts support Révérend's diagnosis of fatal tuberculosis? On the positive side, General Bolívar succumbed to an illness with many of the cardinal features of galloping consumption (fever, productive cough, and cachexia [profound weight loss]). Even more compelling are the autopsy findings of lungs riddled with tubercles (areas of chronic inflammation typical of tuberculosis but also other chronic infections) and cavities. Nevertheless, if Bolívar did die of far-advanced cavitary tuberculosis, possibly with laryngeal involvement, as indicated by his terminal hoarseness, he would have been extraordinarily contagious. If so, how did Révérend, who lived to the ripe old age of 85, escape infection (33)—as well as Manuela Sáenz, the General's longtime mistress, who apparently died of diphtheria, not tuberculosis, at age 60 (35), and also his nephew, Fernando, who was his uncle's private secretary and confidant throughout his terminal illness and lived to age 88 (36)? Why were episodes of hemoptysis not prominent? If Bolívar's lungs were contaminated by the little kisses he received from his mother, as long maintained (37), how did his two sisters and brother all escape a similar fate? Perhaps most important, the chronic cavitary form of pulmonary tuberculosis and the disseminated form rarely coexist. If this is true, as reflected in numerous case series of the latter (38–40), how does one explain the presence of pulmonary cavities and evidence of simultaneous invasion of the brain, liver, and mesenteric glands on post-mortem examination?

If Bolívar's fatal illness was not tuberculosis, what was it? Of the myriad possibilities (41) (Table 7.1), which might be explored in tests performed on specimens recently removed from the General's casket in the National Pantheon in Caracas (see below) (42–44), two are of particular interest—arsenicosis (chronic arsenic intoxication) and paracoccidioidomycosis (a progressive fungal infection indigenous to South America) (41).

Bolívar's headaches, weakness, apathy, abdominal pain, enlarged liver (hepatomegaly), pulmonary complaints, coarse dark skin, and cachexia are all consistent with, though certainly not diagnostic of, arsenicosis (Table 7.2) (45, 46). Arsenic-based remedies were popular in Bolívar's day following the introduction

TABLE 7.1

Diagnostic Considerations and Potential Tests to be Performed on Bolívar's Remains

Possible Diagnoses	Cause	Test
INFECTIONS		
Tuberculosis	*Mycobacterium tuberculosis*	PCR or electron microscopy
Paracoccid-ioidomycosis	*Paracoccidioides brasiliensis*	"
Histoplasmosis	*Histoplasma capsulatum*	"
Melioidosis	*Burkholderia pseudomallei*	"
Syphilis	*Treponema pallidum*	"
Bacterial pneumonia	*Haemophilus influenzae*	"
	Haemophilus spp.	"
	Streptococcus pneumoniae	"
	Staphylococcus aureus	"
	Klebsiella spp.	"
	Pseudomonas aeruginosa	"
TOXINS		
Arsenicosis	Arsenic	Inductively coupled plasma mass spectrometry
Cantharidin intoxication	Extract from *Lytta vesicatoria*	Gas chromatography mass spectrometry
GENETIC OR ACQUIRED		
Diabetes mellitus	Insulin deficiency or resistance	None
Hemochromatosis	Genetic iron overload	PCR mutational analysis, tissue iron analysis
Wilson's disease	Genetic copper overload	Tissue copper analysis
Adrenal insufficiency	Steroid hormone deficiency	None
Familial Mediterranean fever	Autosomal recessive disease	PCR mutational analysis
Lung tumor	Cancer	Computed tomography of bony remains for metastases
Cardiac tumor	Cancer	Computed tomography of bony remains for metastases
Epilepsy	Seizure disorder	None

PCR, polymerase chain reaction.
Adapted from reference 41.

TABLE 7.2

Clinical Features of Chronic Arsenic Intoxication Among 156 Cases Diagnosed in West Bengal

Symptoms	No. (%) of Cases	Signs	No. (%) of Cases
Weakness	110 (70.5)	Pigmentation[6]	156 (100.0)
Headache	32 (20.5)	Keratosis[6]	96 (61.5)
Burning eyes	69 (44.2)	Anemia	74 (47.4)
Nausea	17 (10.9)	Hepatomegaly[7]	120 (76.9)
Abdominal pain	60 (38.4)	Splenomegaly[8]	49 (31.4)
Epigastric[1]	39 (25.0)	Ascites[9]	5 (3.0)
Periumbilical[2]	21 (13.4)	Pedal edema[10]	18 (11.5)
Diarrhea	51 (32.6)	Abnormal lung exam	45 (28.8)
Cough	89 (57.0)	Polyneuropathy[11]	21 (13.4)
Productive	53 (33.9)		
Nonproductive	36 (23.1)		
Hemoptysis[3]	8 (5.1)		
Dyspnea[4]	37 (23.7)		
Paresthesia[5]	74 (47.4)		

[1]Upper abdominal, [2]mid-abdominal, [3]bloody sputum, [4]shortness of breath, [5]tingling, numbness, or pain, [6]dark or horny areas of skin, [7]enlarged liver, [8]enlarged spleen, [9]abdominal fluid, [10]swollen feet, [11]multiple dysfunctional peripheral nerves.
Adapted from reference 45.

in the 1770s of Fowler's solution, a potassium arsenate-containing medicinal used to treat malaria, syphilis, and many other ailments. As noted above, Bolívar's recurrent attacks of "biliary fever" (probably malaria) were treated with an arsenic-based medicine, though the particular one given to him is unknown. He likely was exposed to additional arsenic in the food and water he consumed while campaigning in the Andes, where high levels of the element have been detected in soil and also the tissues of pre-Colombian mummies buried there (47, 48).

Bolívar's complexion, as noted above, changed from white as a youth to dark and rough 3 years before he died. This transformation might simply have been the result of years of exposure to the harsh elements during his campaigns. However, it's also possible that it was an additional manifestation of arsenicosis, in that diffuse melanosis (hyperpigmentation), papules (nodules), and keratoses (horny patches) are among the earliest cutaneous manifestations of such intoxication (49). In present-day Bangladesh, arsenic contamination of drinking water has been closely linked to such skin changes (50). Interestingly, facial flushing, which Bolívar manifested during episodes of "biliary fever," is a reaction to arsenic tonics that practitioners of Bolívar's day regarded as desirable (51). Peripheral neuropathy manifested by focal burning, tingling, or weakness or paralysis is another complication of arsenicosis, which Bolívar apparently did not develop.

Arsenic intoxication also might have contributed to the General's pulmonary difficulties, the onset of which coincided with and were likely precipitated by an attempted assassination—just one of several—in 1828 (52). Bolívar was in Lima at the time. To escape his attackers, he spent 3 hours shivering under a bridge in the murky water of the San Agustín River. Shortly thereafter, his respiratory difficulties flared. The clinical and pathological characteristics of his pulmonary disorder are typical of a refractory bacterial pneumonia that degenerated into nontubercular bronchiectasis—a process that evolves over months to years and manifests as productive cough, fatigue, dyspnea, and weight loss. Moreover, it is a disorder easily confused with tuberculosis (53, 54). If Bolívar's green pericardial fluid was indicative of a purulent pericarditis, likely it would have been caused by bacteria spreading from preexisting bronchiectasis—a dreaded complication of such infections before the advent of antibiotics (55).

Chronic arsenic exposure, for reasons not entirely clear, predisposes to both bronchiectasis and cancer (56, 57). The latter complication of arsenicosis, one that is epidemic in present-day Bangladesh (50), might explain Bolívar's hoarseness (due to paralysis of the left recurrent laryngeal nerve) and, if metastatic to the liver and abdominal lymph glands, also his yellow countenance terminally, his enlarged liver, and his "obstructed mesenteric glands." His terminal hematuria, too, might have been due to metastatic cancer. However, more likely it was due to a low-grade coagulopathy (clotting disorder) caused by the cathardin-based blistering plasters administered by Dr. Révérend (58). His chronic constipation was atypical of chronic arsenicosis, which generally is associated with diarrhea rather than constipation (45) (Table 7.2).

Bolívar's physician's had no effective treatment for arsenicosis. Today patients are given binding agents (chelators), which by increasing the water solubility of arsenic promote its urinary excretion. Vitamin A is also used to treat the skin problems associated with chronic arsenic intoxication. Unfortunately, none of the treatments currently available have been shown to relieve the serious complications of chronic arsenicosis (45).

Paracoccidioidomycosis, although not a perfect fit, in certain respects is an even better explanation for the clinical, epidemiological, and pathological facts of Bolívar's case. In fact, it might account for nearly all such facts—the fever, the weight loss, the apathy, the hoarseness, the productive cough, the flank pain, the skin changes, the thready pulse, the heightened sense of smell, the hematuria, the absence of secondary cases of the infection, and the presence of both cavitary pulmonary disease and disseminated granulomatosis (extrapulmonary spread of the infection) in the same patient (59–66).

Paracoccidioidomycosis, also known as "South American blastomycosis", is a fungal infection caused by *Paracoccidiodes brasiliensis*, and one of the most common deep-seated mycoses (systemic fungal infections) of tropical Latin America. Although Brazil has the highest number of cases, the infection is endemic throughout much of the region in which Bolívar campaigned. Unlike tuberculosis, with which it is all too often confused, paracoccidioidomycosis is not transmitted from person to person. Therefore, whereas Bolívar would likely have passed on his infection to intimate contacts if he had had fulminant tuberculosis, he would not have done so if he had died of paracoccidioidomycosis. Soil is believed to be the microbe's natural habitat and its portal of entry into the body, the lungs. The disease has a long latent period (the time elapsing between invasion by the microbe and the first signs of illness caused by the microbe), rarely manifesting clinically before the age of 30. Men are affected 15 times more often than women (66).

In advanced cases of paracoccidioidomycosis, unlike those of tuberculosis, progressive cavitary lung lesions regularly coexist with disseminated foci of infection in sites such as the tongue, liver, mesenteric lymph nodes, and adrenal glands (66). Productive cough is common, hemoptysis less so. Fever and weight loss occur in over half the cases, hoarseness due to laryngeal involvement in a fifth, and hepatomegaly in 18 percent. In the rare instances in which calcified pulmonary nodules have been encountered—as for example the "calcareous concretion about the size of a hazelnut" found by Révérend in Bolívar's lung—they have been attributed to co-infection with either tuberculosis or histoplasmosis (another systemic fungal infection) (60), which occurs in 15 percent of cases (66). Myocarditis (infection involving the heart) has also been observed, though infrequently. Invasion of the adrenal glands is common, occurring in as many as 85 percent of symptomatic adults (66). Seven percent of cases show evidence of Addisonian crisis (acute deficiency of hormones produced by the adrenal glands), such as profound weakness, cold extremities, and the thready pulse exhibited by Bolívar. In the General's case, destruction of the adrenal glands was indicated further by his dark, coarse skin and perhaps also by his heightened sense of smell, a little-known feature of adrenal insufficiency (67). Today we have drugs that are effective against both paracoccidioidomycosis (amphotericin B) and tuberculosis (isoniazid, ethambutol, rifampin, and many others). Bolívar's physicians had no effective treatments to offer the General.

Shortly before midnight on July 16, 2010, Venezuelan President Hugo Chávez and a team of soldiers, forensic specialists, and presidential aides entered the National Pantheon in Caracas, unscrewed the lid of the General's casket, and removed several fragments of bone and some teeth (41–43). These were sent to a newly inaugurated state forensic laboratory for analysis (40). An attempt first will be made to verify the remains as those of "El Libertador" by comparing DNA retrieved from the specimens with that extracted from the bones of Bolívar's sisters, Juana and María Antonia (68). The other tests to be performed have not yet been revealed to the public but presumably will include assays for arsenic, *Mycobacterium tuberculosis*, and *P. brasiliensis*. If and when these analyses have been completed, the challenge will be one of interpreting the results. Almost certainly disputes will arise not just with regard to their meaning but also their validity. For these reasons, Bolívar's second post-mortem examination is not likely to close the book on the etiology of his fatal disorder. In all likelihood, the information contained in the clinical summary provided above and Révérend's autopsy report will remain the principal evidence upon which the solution to the General's medical labyrinth will have to be based.

Arsenic intoxication, in particular, will be difficult if not impossible to prove, even if high levels of the metal are detected in forensic samples. Arsenic levels correlate poorly with symptoms of intoxication. Moreover, it is rarely possible to differentiate external contamination of specimens from elevated levels due to ingested arsenic. Similar questions will arise if Chávez's investigation finds *P. brasiliensis* in specimens taken from Bolívar's tomb, since the fungus is also a potential soil contaminant. *M. tuberculosis* is virtually never a contaminant. Therefore, if it is detected, there will be little doubt that the General was infected by the bacterium but no guarantee that tuberculosis was his only problem, or for that matter his principal medical problem. If neither *P. brasiliensis* nor *M. tuberculosis* is detected, neither infection can be excluded, since their absence might simply reflect the fact that, while they might have invaded Bolívar's lungs, they would not necessarily have also invaded the bones or teeth being examined.

On one of the four faces of an obelisk erected by the city of Cartagena in honor of El Libertador at the time of his funeral is a shield with the inscription *Extinctus Amabitur Idem* ("The same [hated] man will be loved after he's dead") (1). There were those who hated Bolívar while he lived for having widowed so many during his war for independence and for having been no less savage than the other side. When the war ended and 16 million Americans were left at the mercy of tyrants, many blamed him for this, too. As charged by his former chief of staff, Gen. H. L. V. Ducoudray Holstein:

"…he placed under the name of intendants, military chieftains, the greatest part of whom were totally unacquainted with any kind of administration whatever... the finances are so ruined that Bolívar knows not how, any longer, to pay the interest of the English loans and keep the national credit even up to its present sunken state. Thus has he destroyed the welfare of Colombia, and ruined Perú... But the worst of Bolívar's acts is the last, where he has thrown off his flimsy mask and declared that 'bayonets are the best, the only ruler of the nation'." (69)

Bolívar died rejected and alone on his way into exile. However, his fire, which seemed to have extinguished at the time of his death, simply slumbered beneath the ashes. Today the world continues to marvel at the "brilliance of [a] life that would never, through all eternity, be repeated again" (70).

References

1. Révérend AP. *La Ultima Enfermedad, Los Ultimos Momentos y Los Funerales de Simón Bolívar.* Paris: Hispano-Americana de Cosson and Co., 1866:1–35.

2. Shepherd WR. Bolívar and the United States. *Hispanic American Historical Rec* 1918 (August):270–298.

3. Bingham H. On the route of Bolivar's great march. *Geographical Journal* 1908;32(4):329–347.

4. Maruois A. Bolívar et l'opinion Française. *Rev l'Amerique Latine Paris* 1924 (Decembre):554–572.

5. Letter from Bolívar to General Lafayette: on George Washington. March 20, 1826.

6. Marquez GG. *The General in his Labyrinth* (translated by E. Grossman). New York: Vintage Books, 1999:37.

7. Villamarín Pulido LA. *The Delirium of the Liberator.* Bogotá, Colombia: Penclips Publicidad y Deseño, 2006:7.

8. Lynch J. *Simón Bolívar. A Life.* New Haven, CT: Yale University Press, 2006:54–201.

9. Op. cit. Marquez, p. 8.

10. Op. cit. Lynch, p. 2.

11. Ibid., p. 7.

12. Carbonell D. *Psicopatollogia de Bolívar* (Lib. Franco-Espanola, P. Rosier, ed.). Paris, 1916:31–32.

13. Op. cit. Lynch, p. 55.

14. Ibid., p. 20.

15. Ibid., p. 178.

16. Op. cit. Marquez, p. 191.

17. Op. cit. Lynch, p. 235.

18. Ibid., p. 231.

19. Gonzales F. *Mi Simón Bolívar* (Lucas Ochoa, ed.). Bedout, Medellín, 1930:297.

20. Puyo F. *Muy Cerco de Bolívar* (La Oveja Negra, ed.). Bogotá, Colombia, 1988:140.

21. Figuero Marroquin H. *De que Murio Simon Bolivar?* Guatemala: Imp. Galindo, 1969:3.

22. Reales Orozco A. *Bolívar Frente a los Médicos y la Medicina* (Tercer Mundo, ed.). Bogotá, Columbia, 1988:69.

23. Op. cit. Lynch, p. 229.

24. Ibid., p. 186.

25. Butt J. The liberator in defeat. *Times Literary Suppl* 1989 (July):781.

26. Op. cit. Puyo, p. 228.

27. Mackowiak PA. *Post Mortem. Solving History's Great Medical Mysteries*. Philadelphia: ACP Press, 2007:27–82.

28. Fauci AS, Morens DM. The perpetual challenge of infectious diseases. *N Engl J Med* 2012;366:454–461.

29. Op. cit. Lynch, p. 232.

30. Ibid., p. 283.

31. Ibid., p. 273.

32. Ibid., pp. 276–277.

33. Homer. *The Iliad*. Book VIII, l. 443.

34. Schael Martínez G. *El último Médico de Símón Bolívar*. Ed. Concejo Municipal, Caracas: 1983:pp. 34–38.

35. Murray PS. *For Glory and Bolivar: the Remarkable Life of Manuela Sáenz*. Austin: University of Texas Press, 2008:154.

36. Fuentes Carvallo R. Bolívar, Fernando Simón. In Diccionario de Historica de Venezuela, vol. 1, Fudación Polar, Caracas: 1988.

37. Op. cit. Puyo, p. 12.

38. Sahn SA, Neff TA. Miliary tuberculosis. *Am J Med* 1974;56:495–505.

39. Alvarez S, McCabe WR. Extrapulmonary tuberculosis revisited: a review of experience at Boston City and other hospitals. *Medicine* 1984;63:25–55.

40. Kim JH, Langston AA, Gallis HA. Miliary tuberculosis: epidemiology, clinical manifestations, diagnosis, and outcome. *Rev Infect Dis* 1990;12:583–590.

41. Auwaerter PG, Dove J, Mackowiak PA. Simón Bolívar's medical labyrinth: an infectious diseases conundrum. *Clin Infect Dis* 2011;52:78–85.

42. Rondón P. Venezuela exhumes hero Bolivar's bones for tests. *Reuters*, July 16, 2010.

43. Padgett T. Why Venezuela's Chávez dug up Bolívar's bones. Available online at http://time.com/time/printout/0,8816,2004526,00.html.

44. Halvorssen T. Behind exhumation of Simón Bolívar is Hugo Chávez's warped obsession. *Washington Post*, July 25, 2010.

45. Guha Mazumder DN, Das Gupta J, Santra A, et al. Non-cancer effects of chronic arsenicosis with special reference to liver damage. In Abernathy CA, Calderon RL, Chappell WR, eds. *Arsenic: Exposure and Health Effects*. London: Chapman & Hall, 1997:112–123.

46. Sengupta SR, Das NK, Datta PK. Pathogenesis, clinical features and pathology of chronic arsenicosis. *Indian J Dermatol Venereol Leprol* 2008;74(6):559–570.

47. Zaldivar R. Arsenic contamination of drinking water and foodstuffs causing endemic chronic poisoning. *Beitr Pathol* 1974;151(4):384–400.

48. Pringle H. Archaeology. Arsenic and old mummies: poison may have spurred first mummies. *Science* 2009;324(5931):1130.

49. Chowdhury UK, Biswas BK, Chowdhury TR, et al. Groundwater arsenic contamination in Bangladesh and West Bengal, India. *Environ Health Perspect* 2000;108(5):393–397.

50. Arsenic-related mortality in Bangladesh [editorial]. *Lancet* 2010;376:213.

51. Scheindlin S. The duplicitous nature of inorganic arsenic. *Mol Interv* 2005;5(2):60–64.

52. Op. cit. Lynch, pp. 240–242.

53. Blake WC. Should non-tuberculous lung diseases be treated in the tuberculosis sanatorium? *Chest* 1939;5:11–14.

54. Barker AF. Bronchiectasis. *N Engl J Med* 2002;346(18):1383–1393.

55. Parikh SV, Memon N, Echols M, Shah J, McGuire DK, Keeley EC. Purulent pericarditis: report of 2 cases and review of the literature. *Medicine (Baltimore)* 2009;88(1):52–65.

56. Guha Mazumder DN. Arsenic and non-malignant lung disease. *J Environ Sci Health A Tox Hazard Subst Environ Eng* 2007;42(12):1859–1867.

57. Mazumder DN, Steinmaus C, Bhattacharya P, et al. Bronchiectasis in persons with skin lesions resulting from arsenic in drinking water. *Epidemiology* 2005;16(6):760–765.

58. Karras DJ, Farrell SE, Harrigan RA, Henretig FM, Gealt L. Poisoning from "Spanish fly" (catharidin). *Am J Emerg Med* 1996;14:478–483.

59. Marsiglia I, Pinto. Adrenal cortical insufficiency associated with paracoccidioidomycosis (South American blastomycosis). Report of four patients. *J Clin Endocr* 1966;26:1109–1115.

60. Salfelder K, Doehnert G, Doehnert H-R. Paracoccidioidomycosis. Anatomic study with complete autopsies. *Virchows Arch Abt Path Anat* 1969;348:51–76.

61. Restrepo A, Robledo M, Gutierrez M, Sanclemente M, Castañeda E. Calle G. Paracoccidioidomycosis (South American blastomycosis). A study of 39 cases observed in Medellín, Colombia. *Am J Tropical Med Hygiene* 1970;19:68–76.

62. Londero AT, Ramos CD. Paracoccidioidomycosis. A clinical and mycologic study of forty-one cases observed in Santa María, RS Brazil. *Am J Med* 1972;52:771–775.

63. Restrepo A, Robledo M, Giraldo R, Hernández H, Sierra F, et al. The gamut of paracoccidioidomycosis. *Am J Med* 1976;61:33–42.

64. Ferreira MS. Paracoccidioidomycosis. *Pediatr Respir Rev* 2009;10:161–165.

65. Pedroso VS, Vilela C, Pedroso ER, Teixeira AL. Paracoccidioidomycosis compromising the central nervous system: a systematic review of the literature. *Rev Soc Bras Med Trop* 2009;42:691–697.

66. Restrepo A, Tobon AM. *Paracoccidioides brasiliensis*. In Mandell GL, Bennett JE, Dolin R, eds. *Principles and Practice of Infectious Diseases*, 7th ed. Philadelphia: Churchill Livingstone Elsevier, 2010:3357–3363.

67. Henkin R, Barter FC. Studies on olfactory thresholds in normal man and in patients with adrenal cortical insufficiency: the role of adrenal cortical steroids and of serum sodium concentration. *J Clin Invest* 1966;45:1631–1639.

68. http://www.washingtonpost.com/wp-dyn/content/article/2010/08/30/AR2010083004125.html.

69. Holstein HLVD. *Memoirs of Simón Bolívar, President Liberator of the Republic of Colombia and of his Principal General: Comprising a Secret History of the Revolution and the Events Which Preceded it From 1807 to the Present Time.* London: Henry Colburn & Richard Bentley, 1830:269–270.

70. Op. cit. Marquez, p. 268.

8 Old Jack

ALTHOUGH THIS PATIENT was a college professor, a husband, a Sunday-school teacher, and a church deacon, he is remembered most as a soldier who drew his sword for his state and threw away the scabbard (1). He, perhaps more than any commander in history, bewildered his enemies and kept them bewildered (2), giving hope for a brief period to his people that they might prevail in their desperate pursuit of a lost cause. When his light flickered and a week later went dark, only then did it begin to dawn on them that God would let them be defeated (3).

He was a man of stark contrasts, one deeply religious, with unwavering honesty, a powerful sense of integrity, and deep feelings of responsibility, whose ruling maxim as a soldier was "War means fighting and fighting means killing" (4). From the moment he aligned himself with the Presbyterian Church he gave his whole allegiance to living the Christian life (5). And yet, when asked what should be done in response to Northern aggression, he answered simply: "Kill them, Sir! Kill every man!" (6). To petitions for mercy for deserters, his response was no less emphatic: "Is the accused a soldier? Did he desert? If so, he must die!" (7).

His men—boys really—called him "Old Jack," though he was not yet 40 when "a sleep of [Confederate lead] pressed his eyelids down and left them closed for an eternal night" (8). And at the first battle of Manassas, when he rode slowly back and forth along the line—"moving about in the shower of death as calmly as a farmer about his farm when the seasons are good" (9), he earned the sobriquet *Stonewall*, though offensive operations, not defensive stands, were the source of his towering military reputation. He was "an avalanche from an unexpected quarter...a thunderbolt from a clear sky...secretiveness marked [his] every move" (10).

He was a Virginian raised by a series of relatives after losing his alcoholic father to typhoid fever when he was 2 and his mother to pulmonary trouble (presumed tuberculosis) when he was 7. An older sister died of typhoid fever when she was but 6 years old and an older brother of tuberculosis at age 20. Only a younger sister and half-brother survived him, the former to age 85, the latter to age unknown (11). As children, he and his sister clung to one another, at times in near-desperation, in their struggle to survive as orphans. For each, the other was all that remained of the family. However, she detested the cause for which he fought and died, and when civil war erupted, it strained the lifetime of love she had for him (12, 13).

The patient suffered with chronic dyspepsia most of his life, which he treated with an ascetic diet, heavy in every kind of fruit (14). He was obsessed with his health throughout his early manhood, convinced that each of his organs malfunctioned intermittently to the detriment of his vision, hearing, throat, digestion, liver, kidneys, blood, circulation, nervous system, muscles, and joints (15). In 1849, while stationed at Ft. Hamilton in Brooklyn, New York, he complained of "rheumatism", without specifying further the nature of this complaint, as well as eyes "so weak for some months...[he] could not look at objects through the window...and could not look at a candle not even for a second, without pain" (15). The cause of his photophobia (eye pain on viewing bright light), which continued intermittently for several years, was never determined, although many episodes appeared to be associated with stress (15). Writing, he claimed, gave him "pain in his right side" (15).

To counteract these perceived disabilities, the patient dosed himself with a wide variety of medicines and compresses. He inhaled glycerin, silver nitrate, and the smoke of burning mullein. He also ingested a number of ammonia preparations. For a time he imagined that one side of his body was wasting away and sought to remedy the asymmetry by exercising the withered arm and leg with pumping motions each morning (15). To some these complaints amplified a wonderful eccentricity; to others they were symptomatic of an underlying insanity (16).

Not all of the patient's physical complaints were imagined. When he was 17, he had a brief episode of paralysis of unknown etiology (14). In November 1857, when he was 33, he complained to his sister of "an inflammation of the tube leading to the ear and also inflammation of the throat and very painful neuralgia." Three months later, he wrote: "I have nearly, if not entirely, lost the use of one ear, and my throat has been cauterized about twice a week" (17). Examinations and tests by a Dr. Carnochan revealed an inflamed right tonsil, too swollen to be removed safely. Dr. Carnochan pared off just part of the affected tissue, a procedure from which the patient quickly recovered (18). The earache, which recurred in the winter of 1862 and left the patient partially deaf, was almost certainly otitis media (a middle ear infection) related to recurrent tonsillitis. He had an attack of "bilious fever" at age 36, for which he took the water cure (19). War seemed to agree with his health (20). However, at the first battle of Manassas, he was hit by a bullet or piece of shrapnel, which fractured a middle finger (21). The wound became infected but eventually healed completely (22). While campaigning the year before he died, he suffered briefly with fever and exhaustion, had a recurrence of his earache (23), and was battered and bruised as a result of a fall from his horse (24).

The patient entered West Point in September 1842. For 4 years he plodded, persevered, and struggled, ultimately graduating 17th in a class of 59 as a High Private "who had not demonstrated any aptitude for command" (25). He did not smoke or drink intoxicating liquors (26). He married twice, first at age 29, then again at age 33, 3 years after his first wife died of postpartum hemorrhage following the delivery of a stillborn son. His second wife delivered a lethargic daughter, who died shortly after birth of neonatal jaundice. She then gave birth to a second healthy daughter, who lived to age 26 before dying of typhoid fever (27).

Religion was the very essence of the patient's being. He began each important task with a prayer and ended it with his thanks to God (28). Before the war, he "adhered to a perfect system of regularity," in which he arose each morning at 6 a.m. and "retired not a minute later" than 10 p.m. (29). War, however, murdered his sleep. Never again was he the beneficiary of uninterrupted sleep opportunities. While his men slept, he was all activity (30), and when his generalship faltered, sleep deprivation was in no small part responsible (31). War also transformed him from a kind, gentle, and playful family man to one who knew nothing of conviviality and cared little for conversation (32). During the dark days of civil war, J. E. B. Stuart was the only man who could make him laugh—and who dared to do so (33).

The patient was nearly 6 feet tall and weighed approximately 170 lbs. He had dark brown hair, which tended to curl, a fair complexion turned bronze by outdoor life, a high forehead, curved Indian nose, and thin lips. Large blue-gray eyes dominated a face whose natural expression was a combination of thoughtfulness and fatigue (34). His face would twitch convulsively at the onset of battle (35). His frame was solid and erect; his feet were several sizes larger than normal. His general appearance was more that of a well-to-do farmer than a general, one who might pass through a crowd without attracting attention (36).

He fought 20 battles for the Confederacy. Chancellorsville (Fig. 8.1), his last, brought him apotheosis and death. Its prelude occurred in April 1863 when a Union Army under General Joseph Hooker advancing toward Fredericksburg, Virginia, was met by General Robert E. Lee and 42,000 Confederates at the junction of Chancellorsville Turnpike and the Orange Plank Road. Hooker's force consisted of 65,000 men positioned in front of Lee and another 42,000 waiting nearby in the

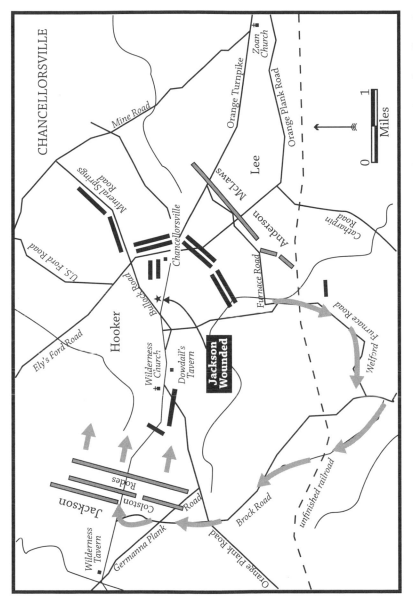

FIGURE 8.1 Map showing the disposition of Confederate (*gray bars*) and Union (*black bars*) forces at Chancellorsville at the time of the patient's celebrated flanking maneuver. (Adapted from Robertson, ref. 37)

city of Fredericksburg. In a radical departure from almost every tenet of military strategy, Lee decided to divide his vastly outnumbered army and attack Hooker's vulnerable western flank. He chose the patient to lead the desperate flanking maneuver (37).

On the early morning of Saturday, May 2, the patient was shivering with what was likely the first sign of a head cold (38). He drank a cup of hot coffee and began the long march toward Hooker's flank. It took him most of the day to get his force of 28,000 troops in position, leaving Lee with only 14,000 men facing Hooker's front. When finally he gave the order to attack at 5:15 p.m., the Federals were taken completely by surprise and began to retreat in near-total disarray. However, night-time intervened before the operation could be completed, and the attack had to be halted just as the Confederates seemed on the verge of destroying Hooker's army (39).

Hoping to mount a night attack and cut off Hooker's northern line of retreat across the Rappahannock, the patient rode out beyond his skirmish line to determine the location and strength of the fractured Union line. As he was returning to his own lines, fighting erupted in the darkness. When shots whizzed in the direction of his mounted party, an aide screamed, "Cease firing! You're firing into your own men!" Major John D. Barry of the 18th North Carolina regiment responded with: "It's a lie! Pour it to them, boys!" In the blaze of fire that exploded from the Confederate line, three bullets struck the patient, two in the left arm and one in the right. The horses stampeded, including Little Sorrel, his horse, which dashed obliquely through the trees toward the Union lines with the patient reeling in the saddle. A tree limb struck the wounded general in the face, knocking off his cap and nearly unseating him before he was able to recover the reins with his injured right hand and bring his horse under control. Captain Keith Boswell and three couriers were killed instantly by the same volley of friendly fire. A. P. Hill's chief of staff, Major H. Palmer, and two other riders were wounded. Three others were captured when their horses raced into the enemy lines (40).

When Captain Richard Wilbourn, a staff officer, reached the patient, he found blood coursing down the general's left wrist into his gauntlet and an unnatural lump in the upper arm. The patient was already so weak and helpless he was unable to remove his feet from the stirrups. When finally lifted gingerly from the saddle, he was too wobbly to stand without support. His left arm was very much swollen but not actively bleeding. It was immobilized with a crude tourniquet fashioned from a handkerchief. A short time later Assistant Surgeon Richard R. Barr appeared with a medical tourniquet, but detecting no hemorrhaging, he elected not to disturb the injured limb. Seeing Federal cannon being unlimbered a short distance away, the officers assisting the patient decided not to wait for an ambulance. When they offered to carry the patient, he insisted on walking though his legs were "rubbery" and his thinking was "foggy." He told his entourage: "If asked who was wounded, just say, 'It is a Confederate officer.'" His bleeding appeared to be minimal at this point (40).

Slowly, step by step, he moved along the Plank Road away from the menacing Union guns, calmly, without uttering so much as a groan. When a litter finally arrived, he was gently laid onto it and raised onto the shoulders of four bearers. They had not traveled more than 40 yards when the Federal artillery began an intense bombardment in their direction. The first round passed over their heads. However, the next round found Private James J. Johnson of the 22nd Virginia Battalion, who was at the left front corner of the litter. When he fell, the patient was pitched to the ground, in all probability on his left shoulder. He groaned in pain (40).

Canister and shell whistled and shrieked through the trees as the general's assistants hurriedly placed him back on the litter and with a new bearer moved as quickly as they could off the Plank Road into the relative safety of the adjacent woods. As they struggled through the dense vegetation, one of the bearers got his foot entangled in a vine and fell. The patient again hit the ground, once again almost certainly on his fractured arm, tearing his brachial artery and triggering heavy bleeding (40).

At about this time, General Dorsey Pender rode up and dismounted. After inquiring about the patient's wounds, he reported: "I will have to retire my troops to re-form them; they are so much broken by this fire." The patient stirred himself from his excruciating agonies, looked sternly at the North Carolina brigadier, and exclaimed in a firm voice: "You must hold your ground, General Pender! You must hold your ground, sir!" (40).

As the little group inched westward away from the menacing artillery in the darkness, the patient grew weaker, with steady hemorrhaging and almost unbearable pain. Several times he asked for spirits, but none was available. Four hundred yards from Plank Road they came to Stony Fork Road, where they met Surgeon William R. Whitehead, who administered a little whiskey mixed with water. An ambulance arrived with two wounded officers already aboard. The weary litter bearers carefully lifted the patient into the crude wagon with metal-rimmed wheels and nonexistent springs. Once the general was aboard, the ambulance lurched along the deeply rutted Stony Fork Road to Dowdall's Tavern, and the attention of the patient's Corps Medical Director, Chief Surgeon Hunter Holmes McGuire (40).

McGuire found his commander's clothes saturated with blood, which continued to ooze from his wounded left arm. He compressed the artery above the wound and then readjusted the crude tourniquet that had been placed by Dr. Wilbourn. The general's skin was clammy, his face pale, and his "thin lips so tightly compressed that the impression of his teeth could be seen through them." Whiskey and morphine (laudanum) were administered. While the wagon pitched and bumped 4 more miles to the Second Corps field hospital at Wilderness Tavern, McGuire kept a finger pressed firmly above the tourniquet to prevent further bleeding (41).

When the wagon reached the field hospital at 11 p.m., the patient was again experiencing chills. After another shot of whiskey he seemed to rally. McGuire informed him that his pulse was hearty enough to permit examination of his wounds under chloroform anesthesia. "If we find it necessary to amputate," he asked, "may we proceed at once?" The patient responded promptly: "Yes, certainly, Doctor McGuire. Do for me whatever you think right" (41).

McGuire was only 27 at the time. He had trained at the Winchester (Virginia) Medical School before transferring to the Jefferson Medical College in Philadelphia, where his father had trained before him. In December 1859, in the midst of the political turmoil surrounding the capture of abolitionist John Brown, he left Philadelphia with a group of Southern students and completed his medical education at the Medical College of Virginia in Richmond. When the Civil War erupted in 1861, he was one of only 27 Southern physicians with surgical experience. Throughout the war, they and their fellow surgeons largely depended on captured Union instruments (such as the amputation kit shown in Fig. 8.2) and

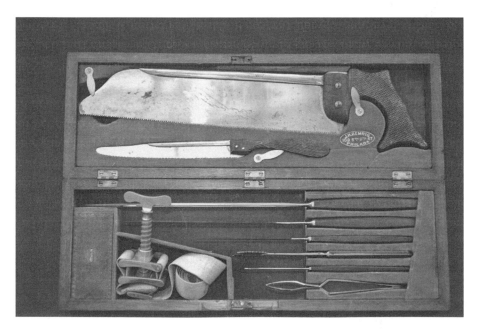

FIGURE 8.2 Amputation kit produced by the J. H. Gemrig Company of Philadelphia during the Civil War. It is typical of ones used by surgeons on both sides of the conflict. This particular kit resides in Davidge Hall at the University of Maryland School of Medicine (photographed with permission).

other medical supplies, such as chloroform, morphine, and quinine, in treating wounded soldiers. McGuire remained with the Confederate Army until the end of the war, when he returned to Richmond and established a busy practice focused on obstetrics, gynecology, and urology. Before his long and distinguished career ended, he served as President of the Richmond Academy of Medicine, President of the Association of Medical Officers of the Army and Navy of the Confederacy, President of the Medical Society of Virginia, President of the American Surgical Association, President of the Southern Surgical & Gynecological Society, and President of the American Medical Association (39).

At a little past 2 a.m. McGuire anesthetized the patient and began his examination. In the right hand, he found a round ball from an old smoothbore musket no longer used by the Federals. It had entered the palm and fractured two fingers before coming to rest just under the skin on the back of the hand. He extracted it easily and gave it to Lieutenant Smith, who later presented it to the patient's wife. McGuire found another bullet wound 3 inches below the left shoulder, a fractured humerus, and a severed brachial artery. A third bullet had entered the left forearm just below the elbow, ripped through the lower arm, and exited above the wrist. He concluded that the limb could not be saved and decided to amputate immediately. Working rapidly with three other surgeons, he sliced through the muscles and tendons with a scalpel and sawed the bone cleanly. As he lifted the limb away, one of his assistants began sealing the blood vessels (41).

McGuire performed a "circular amputation" of the patient's mangled arm. During the procedure, which was standard during the Civil War, a tourniquet was first applied to the injured extremity; the skin was excised in a circular fashion, and the muscles were cut away. The soft tissues were retracted, and the bone was severed more proximally with a saw. Silk, if available, or horsehair was used to ligate vessels. When the amputation was completed, the cuff of skin and soft tissue was drawn back over the stump to function as a cushion. The wound was then covered with a cotton dressing. Although in 1865 Lister demonstrated the capacity of an antiseptic spray (carbolic acid) to prevent surgical infections, the principles of antisepsis and asepsis (sterile technique) were not appreciated, much less practiced, by Civil War surgeons. They routinely performed amputations with unsterile instruments and washed wounds with rags or dirty sponges. They viewed the appearance of pus at the surgical site as "laudable" evidence of normal healing, perhaps because pus indicated the absence of dreaded streptococcal infection—one noted for inflammation without pus. Postoperative complications, such as wound infections, hemorrhage, sepsis, gangrene, and tetanus, were rampant (8). Mortality following amputations of the arm was lower than that after leg amputations. Confederate statistics are unavailable but were probably comparable to those of the Union Army, where of 6,500 patients undergoing upper arm amputations, 1,273 (24%) died (42).

The patient's amputation was completed by 3 a.m. with little additional loss of blood. Isinglass plaster was applied to the facial lacerations he received when hit by the tree limb. Thirty minutes after the operation, he was awakened and given a cup of coffee, his first food in over 24 hours. He slept for a short time before being aroused by his faithful aid, Sandy Pendleton, who briefed him on conditions at the front and asked what should be done. "[The patient] tried to think. He contracted his brow, set his mouth and for a few moments appeared to exert every effort to concentrate his thoughts. For a moment [it seemed] he had succeeded, for his nostrils dilated, his eye flashed its old fire, and his thin lip quivered again, but just for a moment. Presently, he relaxed again, and very feebly, and oh so sadly, he answered, 'I don't know. I can't tell. Say to General [J. E. B.] Stuart that he must do what he thinks best'" (41).

When the patient woke at 9 a.m. on Sunday, May 3, his pain had subsided. He was in good spirits in spite of his amputation 6 hours earlier and felt strong enough to take a little food. He had neither chills nor fever and appeared to be regaining strength rapidly. However, by midmorning he complained of pain in his right side. Although the pain was believed to be the result of an injury incurred when falling from the litter, McGuire "could not discover by examination any evidence of injury. The skin was not bruised or broken, and the lung performed, as far as [he] could tell, its proper function." The pain soon abated (41).

That night the patient slept soundly and awoke Monday morning refreshed and in "admirable condition." General Lee had sent word that the situation at the front was unstable and ordered the patient to be moved as quickly as possible to a safer place. Plans were made immediately to transport him 27 miles further to the rear to Guiney Station. He again was placed in the ambulance and began a 14-hour journey along the Orange Turnpike to the new location. At first he was bright and talkative. However, after the ambulance had bumped and pitched for many miles, he began to feel slightly nauseated. A wet towel placed on his stomach gave him relief (41).

He arrived at the Chandler house in Guiney Station at 8 p.m. It was raining and chilly. He was taken to a small frame house that served as an office, rather than to the noisy main residence, the entire second floor of which was occupied by wounded soldiers. He was laid in a double rope-trellis bed, ate some bread, drank a little tea with evident relish, and drifted off to sleep (41).

The next morning the patient awoke feeling "remarkably well." The stump of his left arm was "covered with healthy granulation" and closing satisfactorily. Although he had no appetite, his attendants were not worried since all of his vital signs were good. He fell asleep that night feeling well. However, at 1 a.m. he awoke nauseated with intense pain in his right side. He asked his attendant to apply a wet towel to his stomach and not to disturb Doctor McGuire, who was sleeping in the next room. The paroxysms of pain intensified. By dawn, every breath produced a piercing sensation in his side. When McGuire finally came to him, he found the patient breathing heavily and occasionally gasping. The general's pulse was rapid. McGuire was convinced that dreaded "pleuro-pneumonia" had developed. He reasoned that the fall from the litter the night the patient was wounded had produced a "contusion of the lung," which was the source of subsequent "inflammation." Heated cups were applied to the patient's chest to draw blood to the surface, and "mercury, with antimony and opium," was administered. Towards evening, the patient felt better, "and hopes were again entertained for his recovery" (41).

Friday, the patient's wounds were dressed again. "The quantity of the discharge from them had diminished, and the process of healing" was progressing satisfactorily. Although the pain in his side had ceased, "he breathed with difficulty and complained of a feeling of great exhaustion." A blistering agent was applied. The next day the patient's breathing was less difficult. However, he appeared to be growing weaker by the hour (41). His wife, who had arrived the day before, thought he was feverish (43).

On Sunday morning

"...his exhaustion increased so rapidly [it was clear to his physicians that]...before the Sun went down, he would be with his Savior....His mind now began to wander, and he frequently talked as if in command upon the field, giving orders in his old way....About half-past one, he was told that he had but two hours to live and he answered...feebly, but firmly, 'Very good, it is all right.' A few minutes before he died, he cried out in his delirium, 'Order A. P. Hill to prepare for action! Pass the infantry to the front rapidly! Tell Major Hawks'—then stopping, leaving the sentence unfinished. Presently, a smile of ineffable sweetness spread itself over his pale face, and he said with an expression, as if of relief, 'Let us cross over the river, and rest in the shade of the trees;' and then, without pain, or the least struggle [the spirit of General Thomas J. "Stonewall" Jackson (Fig. 8.3)] passed from earth to the God who gave it." (41)

The principal source of information concerning Jackson's fatal disorder is a paper published by McGuire in the *Richmond Medical Journal* in May 1866 (41). He wrote his account from memory, since his daily records of Jackson's final days were lost after being captured by Union troops in 1865 (44). Therefore, important details of the general's case summary might be missing from McGuire's paper.

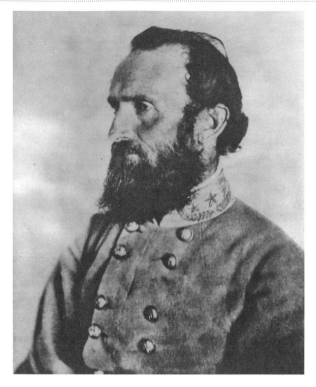

FIGURE 8.3 General "Stonewall" Jackson. "The Chancellorsville photograph" taken 2 weeks before he received his mortal wounds (National Archives).

That being said, based on McGuire's account it seems clear that the dominant features of Jackson's terminal disorder were recurrent, severe pains in the chest accompanied by difficulty breathing and mounting exhaustion and terminal delirium. These developed in the aftermath of profound blood loss from a devastating arm wound and an amputation performed under nonsterile conditions. Although Jackson's wife, Anna, thought her husband was feverish when she arrived 3 days before he died, fever is not mentioned in McGuire's account, nor is cough.

McGuire was convinced that his patient's fatal postoperative complication was "pleuro-pneumonia of the right side." Pneumonia has since been the most widely accepted explanation for Jackson's death (45), in spite of the fact that, according to McGuire's case summary, he never exhibited the two cardinal features of fulminant pneumonia: fever and productive cough. In 1866, the term "pleuro-pneumonia" simply referred to inflammation within the chest affecting both the lung and the adjacent pleuro (the lungs' outer surface) (46). McGuire and his contemporaries had no concept of the role of microorganisms in causing pneumonia or that of inflammation in combating, and sometimes complicating, such infection. Several decades more would have to elapse before the work of Koch, Pasteur, Metchnikoff, and the like elucidating such concepts was generally known and accepted. Therefore, all one might reasonably conclude from McGuire's diagnosis is that he believed the source of his patient's terminal disorder was a destructive process involving the right lung that was simultaneously irritating the adjacent pleura. Although sepsis, gangrene, and tetanus were postoperative complications with which he was no doubt all too familiar, he did not offer any of these as his diagnosis, nor is there anything in his description of Jackson's fatal disorder to suggest that he should have.

McGuire was apparently a careful observer. However, because he had no daily notes to refer to when writing his 1866 article, we can't be certain that Jackson had neither fever nor a productive cough during his terminal illness. If he had, the case for fatal postoperative pneumonia would be enhanced greatly. One then might reasonably propose that Stonewall's "head cold" the morning before he was wounded predisposed him to bacterial pneumonia, which emerged in the post-operative period. However, fulminant pneumonia is a relentlessly progressive, rapidly fatal disorder. It would be atypical in the extreme for an ultimately fatal pneumonia to progress in staccato fashion with two cycles of desperately severe symptoms one day and apparent remarkable recovery the next. Such cycles are characteristic, in fact prototypical, of a different pulmonary disorder—recurrent pulmonary emboli.

Pulmonary emboli are blood clots most often originating in the legs, which dislodge and migrate via the venous system to the lungs, where they come to rest in the pulmonary arteries. They create "difficulty breathing" of the kind experienced by Jackson by infarcting (destroying) areas of the lung fed by the arteries in which they become lodged and by inhibiting oxygenation of blood by a variety of other mechanisms. Jackson likely sustained his first pulmonary embolus at 10 a.m. on Sunday, May 3, approximately 12 hours after being wounded and 8 hours after having had his arm amputated. His risk of deep venous thrombosis (clots developing in the large veins of his legs and also in those of his injured left arm) was extremely high. In a study of major trauma published in the *New England Journal of Medicine* in 1994 (47), the results of which have been corroborated in many subsequent investigations (48–51), 201 of 349 trauma patients (58 percent) were found to have deep vein thrombosis following their injuries. Thirty-nine (11 percent) had clinically suspected pulmonary emboli, and three (0.4 percent) had fatal pulmonary emboli, despite the availability of effective anticoagulants and modern medical care. The average age of patients in the series was 39—Jackson's age at the time of his wounding. Aside from major trauma itself, which has been shown to render the blood hypercoagulable (52, 53), age, need for surgery or blood transfusion, the presence of fractures, especially of the lower extremities, and spinal cord injuries were the principal risk factors for deep vein thrombosis (47). Jackson had many of these risk factors. He was also bedridden postoperatively, yet another important risk factor. During strict bed rest, blood stagnates and all too frequently clots in leg veins because the pumping action of muscles responsible for propelling blood through these veins is markedly reduced during immobilization.

The pain in Jackson's side initially, and then later on, most likely represented peripheral pulmonary infarctions extending to the surface of the lung (the pleura). An irritated pleura is especially painful during respiration because it rubs back and forth against the inner surface of the chest wall as the lungs alternately expand and contract. Because infarctions not extending to the pleural surface are typically painless, Jackson's episodes of chest pain were not by any means necessarily his only instances of pulmonary embolism with infarction.

On the third and fourth postoperative days, Jackson appeared to be recovering nicely. His chest pain had subsided, perhaps because his irritated pleural surface was then being lubricated by inflammatory fluid seeping onto the injured pleural surface. However, on the fifth postoperative day, McGuire found him "suffering great pain . . . of the right side." He also claimed that the earlier episode of chest pain was right-sided. However, if Jackson fell on his left side when dropped from the litter, as reported by one of the attendants with him at the time (Benjamin W. Leigh) (54), McGuire's contention that a "contusion of the lung" was the cause of the initial episode of pain suggests that it was left-sided, not right-sided. If this was the case, and the second episode of pain was correctly reported as right-sided, this would constitute additional support for a diagnosis of recurrent pulmonary emboli, which tend to distribute randomly throughout both lungs.

By the sixth postoperative day, "the pain in [Jackson's] side had disappeared but he breathed with difficulty and complained of a feeling of great exhaustion." If he was having recurrent pulmonary emboli, as his case summary suggests, this would have been when he reached a tipping point with respect to his pulmonary function. By then his lungs likely were so damaged by emboli they were rapidly losing the ability to oxygenate Jackson's blood sufficiently to sustain life. A further reduction in the blood oxygen concentration thereafter due to additional emboli would explain his progressive "exhaustion," then delirium, and finally his death.

No sooner had "death's black cloud enveloped" (55) Jackson then hagiography began replacing historiography. He became "one of the most remarkable soldiers we have ever known" (56), one buried with all of the pomp a grieving capital of the Confederacy could muster for the body of a fallen soldier. His severed arm was interred in the burial plot at Elwood Plantation with its own marker shaded by a small stand of cedar trees surrounded by a knee-high post-and-rail fence. The tiny outbuilding on the Chandler property where he died became a shrine (57).

To be sure, Jackson's success as a Confederate general was out of all proportion to the resources he had at his disposal (58). For many, his were the most shining achievements of the South's military during the period of its greatest prowess (59). "Even Lee's status as the ideal Confederate could not match Jackson's ... for [Jackson] was both a hero and a martyr to the cause, a saint in the eyes of the South, fixed at the right hand of God" (60). Some would even have us believe that if Jackson had survived, the outcome of the war would have been different. Jackson, not Lee, they maintain, had the strategic vision necessary to win key battles and, possibly, the war. If, for example, he had been able to mount his night assault at Chancellorsville, Hooker's army could have been trapped and destroyed. If his alternate plan of capturing a Northern city at Washington's rear, Philadelphia or Baltimore for example, had been implemented in place of the battle at Gettysburg, the South might have prevailed. If he had been present at Gettysburg, the outcome of that battle would have been different, in all probability a Confederate victory. If the Confederates had triumphed at Gettysburg because Jackson had had the foresight to seize Culp's Hill and Cemetery Ridge before the Federals arrived, surely the South would have won the war as well (61, 62).

Stonewall's death was clearly a turning point in the war and might rightly be regarded as the beginning of the end of the South's lost cause. However, most historians believe that the defeat of the Confederacy was inevitable: the North had far greater numbers of soldiers, a limitless supply of war material, a common cause (preserving the union and ending slavery), and a dedicated leader in Lincoln, who had the will and the ability to prosecute the war to a successful conclusion (63). Although according to the *Richmond Examiner* (64) "Hannibal might have been proud of [Jackson's] campaign in the Valley," his performance during the 7-day campaign was near-catastrophic. How he would have fared against Grant, Sheridan, and the other competent Union generals who emerged after 1863 is open to speculation. He was gone before they arrived in northern Virginia. Because he died before Gettysburg and the war's end, white Southerners never saw him humiliated in defeat or struggling to regain his dignity in civilian life (65). By dying at the height of his career, he remained forever a strong and vibrant symbol of the Confederacy with unlimited, and tragically unrealized, potential (60).

References

1. Wood JH. *The War: "Stonewall" Jackson, His Campaigns and Battles, the Regiment as I Saw Them.* Gaithersburg, MD: Butternut Press, 1984:11.

2. *Philadelphia Weekly Times*, April 7, 1877.

3. Robertson JI, Jr. *Stonewall Jackson. The Man, the Soldier, the Legend.* New York: MacMillan Publishing USA, 1997:755.

4. Ibid., p. xiii.

5. Ibid., p. vii.

6. Chambers L. *Stonewall Jackson*. Vol. 1. New York: William Morrow, 1959:563.

7. French SB. *Centennial Tales: Memories of Colonel "Chester" S. Bassett French*. New York: Carlton Press, 1962:15.

8. Virgil. *The Aeneid*. xii, l. 29, 30.

9. Op. cit. Robertson, p. 263.

10. Ibid., p. xiv.

11. Ibid., pp. 7–10.

12. Ibid., p. 691.

13. Farwell B. *Stonewall. A Biography of General Thomas J. Jackson*. New York: WW Norton & Co., 1992:xi.

14. Op. cit. Robertson, p. 19.

15. Ibid., pp. 85–88.

16. Ibid., pp. 275, 380–381, 418, 438.

17. Ibid., p. 180.

18. Arnold TJ. *Early Life and Letters of General Thomas J. Jackson*. New York: Fleming H. Revell, 1916:265–266.

19. Op. cit. Robertson, p. 203.

20. Ibid., p. 332.

21. Ibid., p. 263.

22. Ibid., pp. 271–272.

23. Ibid., p. 667.

24. Ibid., p. 588.

25. Ibid., pp. 42–44.

26. Ibid., p. 299.

27. Ibid., pp. 147, 157, 183, 760.

28. Ibid., p. x.

29. Ibid., pp. 189–190.

30. Henderson GFR. *Stonewall Jackson and the American Civil War*. New York: Barnes & Noble, 1898/2006:321, 540.

31. Mackowiak PA, Billings FT III, Wasserman SS. Sleepless vigilance. "Stonewall" Jackson and the duty hours controversy. *Am J Med Sci* 2012;343:146–149.

32. Op. cit. Robertson, p. 28.

33. Ibid., p. 235.

34. Ibid., p. 22.

35. Fonderden CA. *A Brief History of the Military Career of Carpenter's Battery*. New Market, VA: Henkel, 1911:20.

36. Hewitt LL. A Confederate foreign legion: Louisiana "Wildcats" in the Army of Northern Virginia. *J Confederate Hist* 1990;6:62.

37. Op. cit. Robertson, pp. 701–727.

38. Ibid., pp. 712, 713.

39. Hanks JB. "You can go forward, the . . .": General Stonewall Jackson and Dr. Hunter McGuire encounter the Federals at Chancellorsville, 1863. *Am Surgeon* 2000;66:515–526.

40. Op. cit. Robertson, pp. 728–736.

41. McGuire HH. Last wound of the late Gen. Jackson (Stonewall)—The amputation of the arm—his last moments and death. *Richmond Med J* 1866 (April):403–412.

42. Op. cit. Farwell, p. 513 f11.

43. Op. cit. Robertson, p. 749.

44. Op. cit. Farwell, p. 522 f3.

45. Op. cit. Henderson, p. xv.

46. Gorham LW. What was the cause of Stonewall Jackson's death? Was it pleuropneumonia, pulmonary embolism or fat embolism? *Arch Intern Med* 1963;111:52–56.

47. Geerts WH, Code KI, Jay RM, et al. A prospective study of venous thromboembolism after major trauma. *N Eng J Med* 1994;331:1601–1606.

48. Gearhart MM, Luchette FA, Proctor MC, et al. The risk assessment profile score identifies trauma patients at risk of deep vein thrombosis. *Surgery* 2000;128:631–640.

49. Knudson MM, Ikossi DG, Khaw L, et al. Thromboembolism after trauma. An analysis of 1602 episodes from the American College of Surgeons National Trauma Data Bank. *Ann Surg* 2004;240:490–498.

50. Schultz DJ, Brasel KJ, Washington L, et al. Incidence of asymptomatic pulmonary embolism in moderately to severely injured trauma patients. *J Trauma* 2004;56:727–733.

51. Van Stralen KJ, Rosendaal FR, Doggen CJM. Minor injuries as a risk factor for venous thrombosis. *Arch Intern Med* 2008;168:21–26.

52. Owings JT, Bagley M, Gosselin R, et al. Effect of critical injury on plasma antithrombin activity: low antithrombin levels are associated with thromboembolic complications. *J Trauma: Injury Infect Crit Care* 1996;41:396–406.

53. Engelman DT, Gabram SGA, Allen L, et al. Hypercoagulability following multiple trauma. *World J Surg* 1996;20:5–10.

54. Op. cit. Robertson, p. 733.

55. Homer. *The Iliad*, xvi, l. 398.

56. Op. cit. Robertson, p. ix.

57. Op. cit. Farwell, p. 513 f13.

58. Op. cit. Henderson, p. 361.

59. Freeman DS. *Lee's Lieutenants. A Study in Command* (One-volume abridgement by S. Sears). New York: Simon & Schuster, Inc., 1889:30.

60. Op. cit. Henderson, p. xvi.

61. Layton TR. Stonewall Jackson's wounds. *J Am Coll Surg* 1996;183:514–524.

62. Mathiasen H. Bugs and battles during the American Civil War. *Am J Med* 2012;125:111.

63. Beringer RE, Hattaway H, Jones A, Still WN. *Why the South Lost the Civil War*. Athens, GA: University of Georgia Press, 1986:4–38.

64. *Richmond Examiner*, May 11, 1863.

65. Op. cit. Henderson, p. xi.

9 Mortal Wound

THIS PATIENT WAS a mongrel—"a mixture of all sorts, as only America brings forth" (1). He was a common man who was yet uncommon, "both steel and velvet, hard as a rock and soft as a drifting fog, who held in his heart and mind the paradox of terrible storm and peace unspeakable and perfect" (2). He had a face so awful ugly that some rated it the ugliest eyes ever beheld (1). Others saw beauty in it emanating from bright dreamy eyes that seemed to gaze through you without looking at you (3). While he lived, he was vilified as an "ape, gorilla, fool, filthy storyteller, despot, liar, thief, braggart, buffoon, usurper, monster, tortoise, ignoramus, old scoundrel, perjurer, robber, swindler, tyrant, fiend, butcher, land pirate" (4), but after he was dead, words could not be found to adequately describe the magnificence of the man or his legacy.

He was never in a college or an academy as a student and didn't study English grammar until he was 23 and a lawyer (5). Even so, when called upon to honor his nation's fallen soldiers, he was as eloquent as Pericles. He had a mind "like a piece of steel—very hard to scratch anything on it, and almost impossible after it was there to rub it out" (6). Though lacking in administrative experience and dismissed as a third-rate Western lawyer and fourth-rate lecturer ignorant of proper grammar (2), he had no superior as a stump speaker (7). When elected president, he was more of an executive than almost anyone expected (8). He told hilarious, self-deprecating stories that made him laugh harder than anyone else, but when circumstances called on him to save the nation from extinction, he was as "cool as death" (9).

He was born on February 12, 1809, in Hodgenville, Kentucky (10). When he was 7, his father moved the family to Indiana, "partly on account of slavery, but chiefly on account of difficulty in land titles" (11). In 1820, they moved again, this time to Macon County, Illinois, where the patient would make his first political speech (12).

His father was shorter than the patient, only 5'9" (13). Unlike his son, he was a churchgoing religious man (14) with little time for books (15). Like his son, he had a talent for reeling off sayings, yarns, and jokes (15). He died in 1851 of unknown cause (14). The patient's mother was of uncertain paternity. He claimed that she was the illegitimate daughter of a well-bred Virginia planter, and that her illegitimacy was the source of his power of analysis, logic, and ambition (16). In October 1818, when he was only 9, she came down with the "milk sickness" and died. The illness induces violent trembling, vomiting, and stomach pains and is caused by drinking milk from cows that have fed on snakeroot (17). A younger brother died in infancy of unknown cause. An older sister lived to age 21 before dying in childbirth (18).

The patient was self-taught, with barely a year of formal schooling (19). However, he knew about hard work—pulling the cross-cut and the whip saw, driving the frower, harrowing, planting, hoeing, and harvesting (20). He knew about sports, too, wrestling in particular, in which he nearly always stood first (21). In his youth, he mastered rafting, house-raising, boating, foresting, hog-butchering, brewing and distilling, storekeeping, and rail splitting. He was a "wild, harum-scarum kind of person, who always had his eyes open to the main chance" (22), teaching himself surveying, law, and then politics. As a lawyer, he was known for making a poor showing before judge and jury if he believed his client was guilty (23).

During the Black Hawk War of 1832, his company of volunteers elected him captain (24). However, when he ran for public office for the first time later that same year, he finished 8th out of 13 candidates (25). Then in 1834, he won his first important political office, a seat in the Illinois state legislature (26). He was 25. He won again in 1836 and was selected Whig floor leader. Ten years after that, he was elected to the U.S. Congress, having spent a total of 75 cents on his campaign (27). That was his last political victory until elected president in 1860.

He was not a religious man in the conventional sense. He studied the Bible closely and knew by heart its texts, stories, and psalms, which he quoted liberally in addresses to juries and in speeches and letters. However, he was never convinced that the Bible was the revelation of God or that Jesus was the son of God (28). He drank just enough whiskey to know he didn't like the taste and that it did neither his mind nor his body any good. He also smoked enough tobacco to know that he didn't care for it either (20).

The patient married the 23-year-old daughter of a prominent Kentucky family when he was 33. She was bright, well-educated, and opinionated and dared to involve herself in his career, tutoring him in the fine points of proper manners and dress (2). When he failed in his quest for political office, she was the one who pushed, prodded, and propped him up (29).

The two couldn't have been more different (29). He thrived on humor; she had none. He grew up in poverty, she in luxury pampered by slaves. She was fastidious and highly organized; he was hopelessly "unmethodical" (30). She was short, plump, and elegant; he, forever rumpled, had the look of a "long-legged varmint...made for wading in deep water" (31). More than once she chased him out of the house, brandishing a broomstick on at least one occasion and on another waving a knife (29). Even so, they shared a deep tenderness that was a source of strength and solace during the dark years of his presidency.

They had four sons; three died prematurely. The second-born died at age 4 of unknown cause, the third at age 10 of an undiagnosed febrile illness (29). The fourth son survived his father, only to die in 1871 at the age of 18, possibly of tuberculosis (32).

The patient admitted to a touch of hypochondria (33). However, he also had real medical problems. When he was 10, he was kicked by a horse and "lay all night unconscious" (34). At the age of 17, his axe glanced off a log he was chopping and nearly took off his thumb (35). When he was 19, he received a gash over his right eye while fighting off robbers trying to steal a boatload of cargo he was taking to New Orleans. It left a scar there for life (36). And at the age of 21, he broke through the ice while crossing the Sangamon River and nearly froze his feet before reaching his destination (12). He also had scarlet fever and malaria and a lifelong problem with constipation (32). And in 1863, during perhaps the worst time of his presidency, he came down with a mild form of smallpox (37).

He was prone to fits of melancholia so profound that he once claimed: "If what I feel were equally distributed to the whole human family, there would not be one cheerful face on the earth" (38). During his worst episodes of depression, he was so overcome that "he never dared carry a knife in his pocket" (39). Many of his relatives suffered with similar mood swings (40). Given these symptoms, he would be diagnosed with a major depressive disorder today, based on criteria delineated in the *Diagnostic and Statistical Manual of Mental Disorders* of the American Psychiatric Association.

The patient was in excellent health when he began his presidency (41). However, he aged rapidly while managing a war greater than himself and the two houses of Congress combined (42). For 4 years he worked day and night with little food or sleep, making hundreds of decisions each day critical to the nation's survival. As the lines grew deeper in his face and his cheeks became more and more sunken (43), he tried to hide his pain with laughter (44). Although he seemed to grow wiser and broader and stronger as difficulties thickened and perils multiplied (45), his life springs were gradually worn away by the burdens of the presidency, and he suspected he wouldn't last beyond the end of the war (46).

He was a wiry, sinewy, raw-boned man, thin through the chest and narrow across the shoulders, having lost nearly 40 pounds after taking office (32). Even so, he possessed great strength and was wonderfully athletic, though he walked by putting his whole foot flat down on the ground rather than landing it first on the heel (47). Only a few months before he died, he gave a demonstration of wood chopping, during which he made chips fly in all directions and finished by holding the heavy axe by the end of its handle at arm's length without flinching (32). He had a dark complexion with coarse black hair and gray eyes (48) and was uncommonly tall, at 6'4", with long, slender fingers, and legs and arms that appeared long for his body (3). These features have generated endless speculation that he had Marfan's syndrome (see Chapter 1 in *Post Mortem. Solving History's Great Medical Mysteries* (49)) and, if not assassinated in 1865, would have died soon thereafter of one of the cardiovascular complications of the disorder (50–56). The controversy might be settled by examining preserved pieces of fabric stained with his blood and/or fragments of his skull in the possession of the federal government for genetic evidence of the syndrome. However, thus far, forensic experts have not been given access to these relics (57).

He often spoke and dreamed about being assassinated, convinced that he would not outlast the rebellion when his work would have been done (58). Prior to his inauguration, he received letters warning him that he would be killed before reaching Washington (9). After he died an envelope with 80 such letters was found among his effects, and although twice while president he had his hat shot from his head by unknown assailants, he deprecated all attempts to guard his life (59).

An assassin's bullet finally found him on April 15, 1865, during a performance of *Our American Cousin* at Ford's Theatre in Washington, DC. It was just one of hundreds of plays he attended as president. Nothing seemed to refresh him more during trying times than immersing himself in a play (2). However, on this particular evening, he was exhausted and would have skipped the performance but didn't want to disappoint people hoping to see him at the theater (60). General and Mrs. Grant were invited to join him but declined. Eleven other dignitaries, including the President's son, also declined for various reasons before a handsome young couple, Major Henry R. Rathbone and his fiancée, Clara Harris, accepted the presidential invitation (61).

The patient's murder was but one of a series of assassinations planned for that evening by a band of conspirators (Fig. 9.1). Twice they had hoped to kidnap the President and take him to Virginia to force a prisoner exchange but were thwarted by a last-minute change in their target's itinerary. Three of the conspirators quit

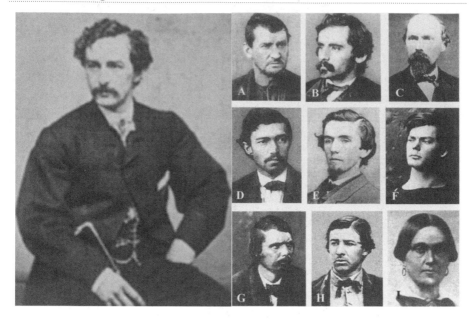

FIGURE 9.1 The assassination team: John Wilkes Booth (left), Edman Spangler (A), Michael O'Laughlin (B), Samuel Mudd (C), Samuel Arnold (D), John Surratt (E), Lewis Powell (F), George A. Atzerodt (G), David E. Herold (H), Mary Surratt (I). (Adapted from reference 62)

in disgust after the failed attempts, but not the ringleader. Learning that the President was to attend the performance of *Our American Cousin* on April 15, he determined to assassinate the patient himself. He assigned one of his coconspirators to murder the Secretary of State and another to shoot the Vice President that same evening. Only the patient's assassination succeeded (62).

The patient was seated in a private box in Ford's Theatre when shot with a .44-caliber bullet fired from a Derringer at close range. The bullet entered the back of his skull to the left of the midline and just above the left lateral sinus (a large venous channel that drains blood from the left side of the brain), which it severed (Fig. 9.2). It penetrated the dura mater (the outermost membrane covering the brain), passed through the left posterior lobe of the brain into the left lateral ventricle, and came to rest in the white matter, just above the anterior portion of the left corpus striatum. It fractured both orbital plates of the frontal bone, causing the orbits (eye sockets) to become engorged with blood and pushing fragments of bone into the brain (63).

Dr. Charles A. Leale, a 23-year-old assistant surgeon, U.S. Volunteers, reached the patient within minutes of the shooting and was accosted immediately by a distraught First Lady crying: "Oh, physician! Is he dead? Can he recover?" The President was not yet dead. However, after a cursory examination, Leale announced: "His wound is mortal; it is impossible for him to recover" (64).

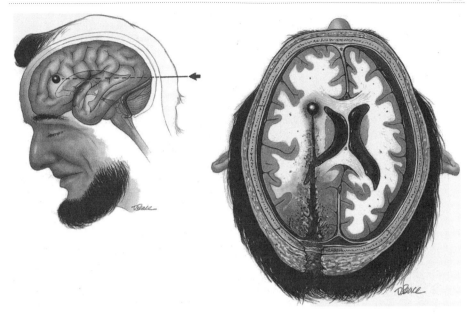

FIGURE 9.2 Artist's depiction of the patient's gunshot wound (*left*) and its damage to the patient's brain as revealed at autopsy (*right*). (From reference 62, with permission from Elsevier)

The President was in a state of general paralysis when Leale reached him; his eyes were closed, and he was deeply comatose. His breathing was intermittent and exceedingly stertorous (consisting of harsh snores and gasps). Leale put his finger on the patient's right radial pulse but could perceive no movement of the artery. While placing the President in a recumbent position, his hand came in contact with a clot of blood near the left shoulder. Supposing the patient had been stabbed there, he had his coat and shirt cut away to identify the source of the hemorrhage. Finding no wound near the shoulder, he began examining the patient's head and soon passed his fingers over a large firm clot of blood situated about 1 inch below the superior curved line of the occipital bone at the back of the skull and 1.5 inches to the left of midline. He removed the coagula (clot) easily and passed the little finger of his left hand through the perfectly smooth opening made by the ball that had entered the brain. As soon as he removed his finger, a slight oozing of blood followed, and the patient's breathing became more regular and less stertorous. Leale then placed a small quantity of brandy and water in the President's mouth, which passed into the stomach and was retained (65).

Shortly after 10 p.m., less than 20 minutes after being shot, the President was transported to the house of a Mr. Peterson, opposite Ford's Theatre. His clothes were removed; he was covered with blankets; and bottles of hot water and warm blankets were applied to his legs and abdomen in an effort to stimulate his circulation. A slight ecchymosis (bruise) was present on his left eyelid, and the pupil of that eye was slightly dilated, whereas the right pupil was contracted. Around 11 p.m., the right eye began to protrude, and the ecchymosis increased in size until it encircled and then extended beyond the orbit. The wound at the back of the president's head was kept open by repeatedly inserting a silver probe into it. Around 2 a.m., when the wound was probed to a distance of approximately 2.5 inches, the instrument came in contact with a foreign substance. This being passed easily, the probe was introduced several inches further, when it again touched a hard substance, at first supposed to be the ball. However, when the bulb of the probe was withdrawn and examined, it had no mark of lead, leading the attendants to conclude that the hard substances encountered were pieces of loose bone. The probe was again introduced. This time, the attendant was convinced he encountered the ball. Nothing further was done with the wound except to keep the opening free from coagula, which if allowed to form and to remain for a very short time produced signs of increased compression of the brain. The breathing became profoundly stertorous and intermittent and the pulse more feeble and irregular (65).

Before midnight, the pulse ranged from 40 to 64/minute; the respirations were loud and stertorous at a frequency of about 24/minute. At 1 a.m., the pulse suddenly increased to 100/minute, but soon diminished gradually until 2:54 a.m., when it became barely perceptible. By 6:40 a.m., the pulse was intermittent, with two or three beats felt, followed by an intermission, when not the slightest movement of the artery was perceptible. The inspirations were short and the expirations prolonged, labored, and accompanied by guttural sounds. At 6:50 a.m., the respirations ceased for some time, and then there was a prolonged inspiration, followed shortly thereafter by a sonorous expiration. At 7:20 a.m., Abraham Lincoln (Fig. 9.3), 16th president of the United States of America, breathed his last, and his spirit fled to God who gave it (65).

Why Lincoln died is no mystery. His wound, as Dr. Leale predicted, was mortal, because in 1865 little could be done for patients with such wounds. Today modern advances in trauma care have greatly expanded our capacity to manage traumatic brain injuries and have radically altered the prognosis of patients with injuries like Lincoln's. Could these techniques have saved Lincoln if they had been available in 1865, and if so, what would he have been capable of in the aftermath of such care? These questions were addressed in 2007 by Dr. Thomas M. Scalea, director of the R. Adams Cowley Shock Trauma Center, the world's oldest such center, at the University of Maryland School of Medicine, during the school's bicentennial celebration (66). Dr. Scalea believes that the trauma care discussed below would not only have saved Lincoln's life but would also have restored much of the President's neurological function.

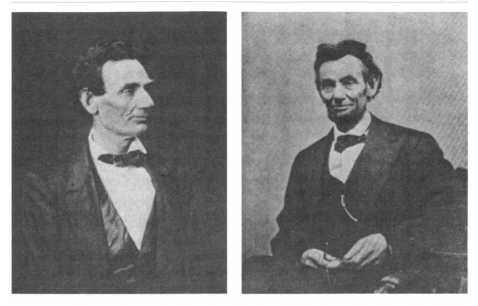

FIGURE 9.3 An 1860 photograph of Lincoln taken shortly before being elected president (*left*) and another taken in 1865 a few days before his assassination (*right*). According to John Hay, the later photograph has "a look as of one on whom sorrow and care had done their worst without victory." (From reference 62, with permission from Elsevier)

Lincoln was shot in the left occiput at close range with a relatively low-velocity bullet. Two young physicians, Dr. Charles Leale, who had graduated from medical school only days before the shooting, and Dr. Charles Taft, just 30 years old, cared for Lincoln. In accordance with the medical practice of the day, they repeatedly probed the President's wound to prevent blood from accumulating within the skull and compressing his brain. For a time, this maneuver relieved Lincoln's respiratory distress.

Lincoln's initial symptoms and his dilated left pupil were caused by cerebral herniation—displacement and compression of vital areas of the brain by blood and edema fluid accumulating within his skull. His physicians remarked that "as long as bleeding continued, the President's condition remained stable. When the flow stopped, the vital signs weakened...It would produce signs of increased compression. The breathing became stertorous and intermittent, and the pulse became more feeble and irregular" (67). As illustrated in Figure 9.2, the most likely path of the bullet that killed Lincoln was through the left lateral sinus. As it traveled through the brain, it created pressure waves that damaged the brain stem (the upper spinal cord). It also produced intraventricular hemorrhage (bleeding into the inner cavities of the brain), a deep laceration of the left cerebral hemisphere, and bilateral subdural hematomas (pools of blood collected on the surface of the brain). In time, these primary injuries (i.e., those occurring at the time of impact) were likely magnified by inadequate delivery of oxygen to the brain resulting from repeated episodes of hypotension and the president's irregular breathing. This, in turn, caused pressure within the skull (the intracranial pressure [ICP]) to rise, producing additional (secondary) damage to the brain (68).

Lincoln's intracerebral hemorrhaging would have caused his ICP to soar. Whereas repeated probing of his wound allowed blood to escape from his skull and for a time relieved his elevated ICP, it also contributed to substantial blood loss. The brain is an extremely vascular organ and when injured bleeds profusely. In fact, Lincoln's attendants commented that his sheets were crimson and his bed surrounded by a pool of blood. Thus, it is likely that he died because of both cerebral herniation and massive hemorrhaging (66).

Modern trauma care involves a continuum of activities that can be artificially divided into several phases. The process begins with a preliminary assessment of the patient at the scene of the injury and application of stabilization measures, such as assisted respiration and the administration of intravenous fluids. Appropriate patients are then quickly transported to trauma centers for specialized care. At the trauma center, another examination is performed to identify immediately life-threatening injuries, which are dealt with as discovered. Next, resuscitation measures as, for example, blood transfusions in the case of Lincoln, are administered as needed, followed by a more systematic, head-to-toe physical examination and appropriate radiographic studies, after which definitive care is given (66).

Today, a trauma system of this sort would be activated promptly if the President were injured. In fact, whenever the President leaves the White House, area trauma centers are alerted so that they are available immediately in case of illness or injury involving the chief executive. When the President travels in Maryland, the Shock Trauma Center at the University of Maryland is the one alerted and remains on standby, ready to provide care as needed (66).

Although the advantages of stabilizing trauma patients in the field, so-called "stay-and-play", versus immediate transport to a trauma center, so-called "scoop-and-run", might be debated in injuries as severe as Lincoln's, there is no question that in an urban environment such as the Baltimore/Washington, DC area, with its trauma center literally just minutes away, the "scoop-and-run" option is the best. One might argue, for example, that patients with brain injuries of the magnitude of Lincoln's should be intubated (have a tube inserted into their trachea to assist ventilation and also to protect their lungs from regurgitated stomach contents) in the field. However, in a recent survey of patients with severe brain injuries treated in the Maryland Trauma System, an organization with considerable airway-management experience, patients intubated upon arrival at the trauma center had a substantially better outcome than those intubated in the field (69). Therefore, Lincoln would have been managed best initially by inserting an intravenous line, through which fluids and blood might be administered, and by assisting his breathing using a ventilation bag attached to a ventilation mask. Once he arrived at the Trauma Center, an endotracheal tube would have been inserted promptly into his upper airway by a trained anesthesiologist (66).

Although hyperventilation (rapid forced ventilation) has traditionally been used to reduce brain swelling in patients with severe head injuries, it has not been shown to improve outcome (70). Hyperventilation does reduce ICP but, unfortunately, does so by diminishing the flow of blood to the brain, which, in turn, reduces the amount of oxygen delivered to the brain. Nevertheless, in patients like Lincoln with impending herniation, hyperventilation is sometimes the only way of lowering ICP rapidly enough to prevent herniation.

President Lincoln's dilated left pupil reflected impending herniation and would have been treated initially with intravenous hypertonic saline solution (a concentrated salt solution) to support his blood pressure and also to lower his ICP by drawing edema fluid from his damaged brain back into the bloodstream. Because Lincoln's ICP was almost certainly extremely high, he also would have been treated with modest hyperventilation. A chest x-ray would have been performed, along with an array of routine blood tests. After a third physical examination searching for previously unrecognized injuries, he would have been rushed to the computed tomography (CT) scanner for a definitive examination of his head injury (66).

In that acute subdural hematomas must be evacuated promptly in patients with signs of impending herniation, Lincoln would next have been wheeled into the operating room for an emergency craniotomy, ideally within 15 minutes of his arrival in the Trauma Center. His surgery would have been performed by neurosurgeons continuously on call in a room permanently on standby for such emergencies. The neurosurgeons would evacuate the President's hematomas, débride the bullet's entrance wound, and repair the damaged dura. They would also place catheters inside his skull to monitor his ICP, cerebral blood flow, and brain oxygen levels, as well as to remove cerebrospinal fluid as needed to lower the ICP. Another head CT scan would be performed looking for evidence of further secondary damage requiring additional surgery. When all necessary surgery had been performed, the president would have been moved to an intensive care unit (66).

Traumatic brain injury, even if unaccompanied by other injuries, is a systemic disorder in that it activates a neurohumoral cascade (a sequence of pathophysiological reactions involving hormones as well as nerves) capable of causing dysfunction of virtually every organ system. The circulatory system and the lungs are especially hard hit. In certain cases, a full-blown systemic inflammatory response ensues, resulting in intestinal dysfunction, renal failure, and a generalized capil-lary leak. Sometimes, patients develop a coagulopathy (inappropriate clotting of the blood), both as a consequence of clotting mediators released by injured brain tissues and as a complication of transfusions given to replace blood lost as a result of both the injury and surgery (66).

While in the intensive care unit, Lincoln's ICP, blood pressure, and blood oxy-gen level each would be monitored closely, with measures taken to optimize the flow of blood and oxygen to his damaged brain. Antibiotics would be given to prevent infection, along with anticonvulsants to prevent seizures. Because trau-matic brain injuries are associated with substantial tissue breakdown, not just at the site of the injury but throughout the body, early intravenous nutritional sup-port would be added to his treatments to facilitate healing. Sequential compres-sion devices would be applied to his legs as soon as he was stabilized, along with low-molecular-weight heparin on the third postoperative day to prevent blood clots from forming in the deep veins of his legs (66).

Some trauma patients develop dangerously high ICPs that are refractory to the measures listed above and require additional, more aggressive interventions to bring their ICP under control. One such intervention is decompressive craniec-tomy, in which a portion of the skull is removed and saved for possible replace-ment at a later date to permit the brain to swell unimpeded in the immediate aftermath of the injury. Because the skull is a rigid container, swelling of the brain or bleeding into it causes the ICP to increase. If it rises to a level greater than the pressure within the brain's blood vessels, blood flow to the brain ceases. In such cases, decompressive craniectomy may be the only effective means of lowering the ICP and restoring proper delivery of glucose and oxygen to the brain. In the R. Adams Cowley Shock Trauma Center, decompressive craniectomy has been used successfully to relieve refractory traumatic intracranial hypertension 80 percent of the time, and achieved a survival rate of 78 percent with a favorable neurological outcome in 50 percent of such patients (71).

The ICP correlates closely with the pressure inside both the thorax and the abdo-men in patients with severe head trauma (72), in all likelihood because of commu-nication between the three anatomical compartments via their venous systems. On occasion, harnessing this relationship is the only means, albeit a drastic one, of alle-viating refractory intracranial hypertension in patients with severe head trauma. In a recent series of 17 such patients, abdominal decompression (opening the abdomen surgically to reduce intra-abdominal pressure) lowered ICP by nearly 50 percent, even in the absence of elevated intra-abdominal pressure preoperatively (73, 74).

Optimal management combining early mobilization, a multidisciplinary approach to treatment, and early aggressive rehabilitation might have saved Lincoln.

However, it could not have restored his neurological function to normal. At best, he would have been left with several permanent neurological deficits. Patients surviving injuries like his tend to have increased impulsivity, lack of emotional control, decreased problem-solving ability, and impaired eye–hand coordination. Given the nature and extent of Lincoln's injury, almost certainly he also would have been left with right hemiplegia (paralysis of his right side) and homonymous hemianopsia (blindness in the right half of the visual field of both eyes), as well as dyslexia, dysgraphia (difficulty writing), and dysphasia (difficulty speaking). However, because his frontal lobe was largely spared, his cognition likely would have remained reasonably intact. His rehabilitation would have been long and difficult and at a minimum would have involved a team of professionals consisting of a physiatrist, a neuropsychologist, a speech therapist, a physical therapist, and an occupational therapist. The full extent of his recovery would have taken several years of intensive rehabilitation to have been realized (66).

When Lincoln died, he was succeeded as president by Andrew Johnson, a Southern Democrat lacking in diplomatic skills and incapable of compromise. Johnson vetoed unsuccessfully many of the civil rights bills Lincoln would have endorsed. He also ignored passage of "black codes" by Southern states, whereby blacks were prevented from leaving current positions or owning land. He tried to force provisional governors to turn over state control to former Confederate leaders and vetoed legislation creating both the Freedmen's Bureau, which was trying to help newly liberated blacks assimilate into a free society, and the Civil Rights Act of 1866. He also vetoed three Reconstruction acts designed to give blacks the right to vote, before Congress finally passed the 14th Amendment in 1868 (75–78).

If Lincoln had lived but been disabled, the situation might well have been even more chaotic, because in 1865 no provision existed for the Vice President or anyone else to take over as chief executive for an incapacitated president. At that time, the Constitution contained provisions for the transfer of such power only when a president died. Not until 1967 was the 25th Amendment passed, which specifies the procedures by which the government deals with an incapacitated president (66) (see Appendix).

Given the extent of the damage to Lincoln's brain caused by the bullet from Booth's Derringer, one would be inclined to dismiss Dr. Scalea's prediction regarding what his team might have accomplished as overly optimistic. However, the case of U.S. Representative Gabrielle (Gabby) Giffords seems to suggest otherwise. On January 27, 2011, she was shot in the head with a Glock semiautomatic pistol. A 9mm bullet entered the back of her head just to the left of the midline at almost exactly the same spot at which Booth's bullet entered Lincoln's head, and traveled the same path as Booth's bullet before exiting through the front of her skull near her left eye socket (Fig. 9.4). Giffords was treated according to a protocol similar to that outlined above, including removal of a portion of her skull to allow her brain to swell unimpeded, after which she participated in an intensive rehabilitation program. Now, a little over a year later, she can walk, she can speak in a halting manner, and she is apparently hopeful of one day returning to politics (79–81).

Although Giffords' case seems to validate Dr. Scalea's conclusions, no two head trauma cases are identical. Whereas Lincoln's and Giffords' injuries have much in common, they also differ in several important aspects. Lincoln was shot with a .44-caliber low-velocity bullet, Giffords with a 9mm high-velocity bullet. Lincoln's bullet didn't exit the skull; Giffords' did. Most important, Giffords' bullet traveled only through the left side of her brain. Lincoln's is thought to have done so as well; however, Leale's description of a bulging *right* eye suggests that the bullet actually crossed the midline into the right cerebral hemisphere, in which case Lincoln's chances of surviving his injury, even if treated in a modern shock trauma center, much less recovering neurological function to Giffords' degree, would be minimal.

On January 4, 2006, Ariel Sharon, then Prime Minister of Israel, suffered a different though no less devastating brain injury—a massive stroke. The Israeli heath care system, arguably one of the best in the world, reacted quickly and decisively with a series of sophisticated interventions, hoping for the kind of miraculous recovery sometimes seen in such patients. In spite of a host of aggressive measures, including several surgeries related to his comatose state, Sharon never regained his cognitive abilities. He was placed in a long-term care facility on November 6, 2007. Six years later, he is alive but in a persistent vegetative state.

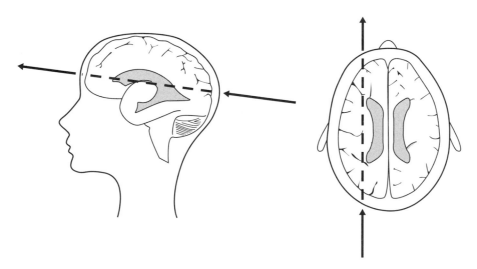

FIGURE 9.4 Path taken by a bullet through Rep. Giffords' brain as reported by the *Guardian* on January 10, 2011.

Abraham Lincoln suffered his massive brain injury almost a century and a half earlier. The health care system in which his physicians operated was far less sophisticated than that of modern-day Israel or the R. Adams Cowley Shock Trauma Center. It had neither the knowledge nor the tools to save Lincoln's life, much less preserve his cognitive abilities, in the aftermath of Booth's attack. If Dr. Scalea's team had had access to Lincoln at the time of the assassination, perhaps he might have survived, albeit with right-sided hemiplegia and homonymous hemianopsia, along with persistent dyslexia, dysgraphia, and dysphasia. If so, he might yet have retained enough cognitive and communicative function to have restrained the forces of prejudice and vindictiveness that marred Johnson's period of reconstruction. Lincoln's genius, after all, was that "In the cave of winds in which he saw history in the making, he was more a listener than a talker" (82).

However, in medicine as in politics, nothing is certain. Although under the care of a trauma team like Dr. Scalea's Lincoln might have made a recovery as miraculous as that of Giffords, he might also have fared no better, or even worse, than under the care of Doctors Leale and Taft. As in the case of Ariel Sharon, modern technology produces tragic failures along with spectacular successes. Sometimes a life is saved only to leave the patient "to linger in dying . . . never again [to] speak, see, hear, or awaken into a conscious being" (83). It is because of such uncertainty that knowing when not to treat can be more difficult and more important than knowing how to treat.

References

1. Sandburg C. *Abraham Lincoln. The Prairie Years and the War Years*. One vol. ed. New York: Harcourt, Inc., 1925:676.

2. Shenk JW. The true Lincoln. *Time* July 4, 2005:38–46.

3. Op. cit. Sandburg, p. 401.

4. Ibid., p. 594.

5. Ibid., p. 179.

6. Ibid., p. 113.

7. Ibid., p. 139.

8. Ibid., p. 257.

9. Ibid., p. 191.

10. Ibid., p. 7.

11. Ibid., p. 9.

12. Ibid., p. 21.

13. Ibid., p. 3.

14. Ibid., p. 107.

15. Ibid., p. 4.

16. Ibid., p. 111.

17. Ibid., p. 11.

18. Ibid., p. 16.

19. Ibid., p. 36.

20. Ibid., p. 15.

21. Ibid., p. 25.

22. Winik J. *April 1865: The Month that Saved America*. New York: Harper Collins, 2001:231.

23. Op. cit. Sandburgp. 79.

24. Ibid., p. 29.

25. Ibid., p. 32.

26. Ibid., p. 41.

27. Ibid., p. 84.

28. Ibid., p. 105.

29. Op. cit. Winik, p. 233.

30. Op. cit. Sandburg, p. 389.

31. Ibid., pp. 92, 157.

32. Lattimer JK. The wound that killed Lincoln. *JAMA* 1964;187:480–489.

33. Op. cit. Sandburg, p. 73.

34. Ibid., p. 12.

35. Ibid., p. 14.

36. Ibid., p. 19.

37. Ibid., p. 448.

38. Ibid., p. 70.

39. Ibid., p. 55.

40. Ibid., p. 47.

41. Ibid., p. 166.

42. Ibid., p. 384.

43. Ibid., p. 259.

44. Ibid., p. 569.

45. Ibid., p. 402.

46. Ibid., p. 606.

47. Ibid., p. 112.

48. Ibid., p. 161.

49. Mackowiak PA. *Post Mortem. Solving History's Great Medical Mysteries*. Philadelphia: ACP Press, 2007:1–25.

50. Rimoin DL, Connor JM, Pyeritz RE, Korf BR, eds. *Emery and Rimoin's Principles and Practice of Medical Genetics,* 4th ed. London: Churchill Livingstone, 2002:3977–4010.

51. Schwartz H. Abraham Lincoln and aortic insufficiency. The declining health of the president. *California Med* 1972;116:82–84.

52. Lattimer JK. Lincoln did not have the Marfan syndrome. Documented evidence. *NY State J Med* 1981;81:1805–1813.

53. Judge DP, Dietz HC. Marfan's syndrome. *Lancet* 2005;366:1965–1981.

54. Kuehn BM. Genes help unravel Marfan pathology, point to potential new therapies. *JAMA* 2005;294:1745–1746.

55. Gelb BD. Marfan's syndrome and related disorders—more tightly connected than we thought. *N Engl J Med* 2006;355:841–844.

56. Kroen C. Abraham Lincoln and the "Lincoln sign." *Cleveland Clin J Med* 2007;74:108–110.

57. Brown D. Lincoln may be 1st recorded case of rare disease. *Washington Post* Nov. 26, 2007:A8.

58. Op. cit. Sandburg, p. 547.

59. Ibid., p. 696.

60. Ibid., p. 704.

61. Op. cit. Winik, p. 221.

62. Friedman WA, Peace D. A gunshot wound to the head—the case of Abraham Lincoln. *Surg Neurol* 2000;53:511–515.

63. Woodward JJ. *Report of autopsy on President Lincoln*, April 15, 1865, original in Surgeon General's office, Washington, DC.

64. Op. cit. Sandburg, p. 711.

65. Leale CA. *The Assassination and Death of Abraham Lincoln, President of the United States*. National Archives of the United States.

66. Scalea TM, Carson SL, Mackowiak PA. Saving President Lincoln. *Am J Med Sci* 2009;337:47–55.

67. Kauffman MN. *American Brutus. John Wilkes Booth and the Lincoln conspiracies*. New York: Random House Publishers, 2005:29, 30, 47.

68. Chesnut RM, Marshall LF, Klauber MR, et al. The role of secondary brain injury in determining outcome from severe head injury. *J Trauma* 1993;34:216–222.

69. Bochicchio GV, Ilahi O, Joshi M, et al. Endotracheal intubation in the field does not improve outcome in trauma patients who present without an acutely lethal traumatic brain injury. *J Trauma* 2003;54:307–311.

70. Muizelaar JP, Marmarou A, Ward JD, et al. Adverse effects of prolonged hyperventilation in patients with severe head injury: a randomized clinical trial. *J Neurosurg* 1991;75:731–739.

71. Aarabi B, Hesdorffer D, Ahn E, et al. Outcome following decompressive craniectomy for malignant swelling following severe head injury. *J Neurosurg* 2006;104:469–479.

72. Saggi BH, Bloomfield GI, Blocher CR, et al. Reversal of intracranial hypertension with acute abdominal compartment syndrome using continuous negative abdominal pressure. *J Trauma* 1998;44:248.

73. Joseph DK, Dutton RP, Aarabi B, et al. Decompressive laparotomy to treat intractable intracranial hypertension after traumatic brain injury. *J Trauma* 2004;57:687–695.

74. Scalea TM, Aarabi B, Bochicchio G, et al. Increased intraabdominal, intrathoracic and intracranial pressure after severe brain injury: multiple compartment syndrome. *J Trauma* 2007;62:647–656.

75. Thomas BP, Hyman HM. Stanton. *The Life and Times of Lincoln's Secretary of War*. New York: Alfred A. Knopf, 1962:392–456, 487, 489, 497.

76. Means H. *The Avenger Takes his Place. Andrew Johnson and the 45 Days that Changed the Nation*. New York: Harcourt, Inc., 2006:226–237.

77. Foner E. *Reconstruction. America's Unfinished Revolution*. New York: Harper and Row, 1988:176–281, 333–346.

78. Benedict ML. *A Compromise of Principle. Congressional Republicans and Reconstruction, 1863–1869*. New York: W.W. Norton, 1974:84–315.

79. Quin B. *Gabrielle Giffords: a political high-flyer*. The Guardian. Jan. 10, 2011.

80. http://articles.cnn.com/2012–01–22/politics/politics_giffords-resigning_1_gabrielle-giffords.

81. http://www.webmd.com/brain/news/20110109/gabrielle-giffords-brain-injury-faq

82. Op. cit. Sandburg, p. 149.

83. Ibid., p. 709.

Appendix

25th Amendment to the Constitution (1967)

Passed by Congress July 6, 1965. Ratified February 10, 1967. Replaced part of Article II, section 1 of the Constitution, originally written in 1783.

Section 1

In case of the removal of the President from office or of his death or resignation, the Vice President shall become President.

Section 2

Whenever there is a vacancy in the office of the Vice President, the President shall nominate a Vice President who shall take office upon confirmation by a majority vote of both Houses of Congress.

Section 3

Whenever the President transmits to the President pro tempore of the Senate and the Speaker of the House of Representatives his written declaration that he is unable to discharge the powers and duties of his office, and until he transmits to them a written declaration to the contrary, such powers and duties shall be discharged by the Vice President as Acting President.

Section 4

Whenever the Vice President and a majority of either the principal officers of the executive departments or of such other body as Congress may by law provide, transmits to the President pro tempore of the Senate and the Speaker of the House of Representatives their written declaration that the President is unable to discharge the powers and duties of his office, the Vice President shall immediately assume the powers and duties of the office as Acting President. Thereafter, when the President transmits to the President pro tempore of the Senate and the Speaker of the House of Representatives his written declaration that no inability exists, he shall resume the powers and duties of his office unless the Vice President and a majority of either the principal officers of the executive department or of such other body as Congress may by law provide, transmit within 4 days to the President pro tempore of the Senate and the Speaker of the House of Representatives their written declaration that the President is unable to discharge the powers and duties of his office. Thereupon, Congress shall decide the issue, assembling within 48 hours for that purpose if not in session. If the Congress, within 21 days after receipt of the latter written declaration, or, if Congress is not in session, within 21 days after Congress is required to assemble, determines by two-thirds vote of both Houses that the President is unable to discharge the powers and duties of his office, the Vice President shall continue to discharge the same as Acting President; otherwise, the President shall resume the powers and duties of his office.

Source: National Archives

10 Voyage to Invalidism

IT'S DOUBTFUL THAT any work, save Newton's *Principia*, ever caused so profound and rapid a revolution in science or made so deep an impression on our thinking as this patient's book (1). It caused us to reevaluate our place among living creatures by laying bare how closely interconnected and endlessly changing is the web of life. Nothing in medicine makes sense today except in the light of his theory. Even personalized medicine, with all of its modern trappings and its use of sophisticated genetic analyses to individualize health care, owes its existence to insights he provided over a century and a half ago (2).

Before this patient developed and published his theory, the myriad species of living organisms that populate our planet were thought to be immutable and fixed. Individual life forms, whether sea anemone, musk ox, or bark beetle, existed as imperfect approximations of a creator's ideal. Individual variations were viewed as irrelevant blemishes, unworthy of study. This patient recognized the critical importance of such variation in determining how we came to be who we are, and why we will not be the same beings indefinitely (4). Because of him, we have come to realize that humans do not stand apart from the rest of biology, as Biblical scripture teaches, but are *literally*, not metaphorically, related to the birds of the air and lilies of the field (2). So revolutionary were these ideas that many considered them, and still do, not just implausible, but immoral and irreligious (3). His ideas shook social convention at its core, which is why, for a time, some considered him "the most dangerous man in England" (2).

And yet, the patient was not by nature an iconoclast, nor did his early years give any intimation of the towering intellect that would enable him to see beyond convention. In fact, the teachers at the Shrewsbury School into whose hands he first fell viewed him as "no better than a dunce" (1). Sports and beetle-collecting were his passion then (1).

When he was 16, he followed in the footsteps of his father, grandfather, and brother and enrolled in Edinburgh as a medical student. Seeing two very badly performed operations, however, cured him of any desire he had of becoming a doctor, and on the advice of his disappointed father, he moved on to Christ College, Cambridge, to pursue a degree in divinity. Although he performed well enough there to graduate, it was a few years later aboard the H.M.S. *Beagle* that his real education took place (1).

The *Beagle* years represented a different kind of school time that lasted 5 years instead of the 2 he had expected. Robert Fitzroy, a grandson of the 3rd Duke of Grafton, was the ship's captain. He had been commissioned by the British Admiralty to survey South America around Tierra del Fuego and back by the West Indies. For the voyage, he required a gentleman companion, naturalist, and savant. John Henslow, a Professor of Botany at Cambridge, knew of the patient's interest in natural history and travel and recommended him for this position. At first the young man's father would not give his permission for his son to join the expedition, fearing the trip would expose him to coarse elements unbefitting a future man of the cloth. A benevolent uncle, however, intervened, won the father over, and on December 27, 1831, the patient departed Plymouth aboard the H.M.S. *Beagle* on what would become one of the great epic voyages of discovery (1).

Before the voyage, the patient's only ailments consisted of an upset stomach "lasting a good many breakfasts" during his teens, and brief eruptions of unknown character of his mouth and hands during his early 20s (4). Over his 5 years aboard the H.M.S. *Beagle* (age 22 to 27), he was seasick whenever the little ship was lively, which, considering the circumstances of the cruise, was more often than not. When he had returned to England and "gastric flatus" made him an invalid, many of his physicians postulated that his *Beagle* seasickness was the cause (5). The patient also had several self-limited fevers, two instances of food poisoning, an inflamed knee and arm, intermittent boils, and heat stroke, all of which resolved without sequelae (6, 7).

In April 1832, while traveling through a Brazilian forest, he began "to feel feverish shivering and...much exhausted, and could eat nothing." He later wrote that he was able to treat himself with cinnamon and port wine, which cured him "in a wonderful manner" (8).

One of his few serious illnesses occurred in September 1834, while he was visiting a gold mine in Chile. His stomach became "disordered" after he drank some Chichi wine. He lost his appetite and became so weak and exhausted he was unable to ride his horse and had to hire a carriage to carry him back to the *Beagle*. This illness lasted nearly 2 months and was never diagnosed. Although the patient doesn't mention fever in his account of the illness, the physician who cared for him dosed him with "a good deal of calomel"—a medication generally prescribed for fevers. The patient believed he had been poisoned by the Chichi wine (9). Others have speculated that the illness was actually an attack of Chilean fever, which quietly festered after an apparent recovery before reemerging years later as a chronic gastric disorder (see below).

The patient returned to England in October 1836 looking very thin but well. For 9 months he made no complaints about his health and gained nearly 16 pounds. His earliest recorded physical complaint was in a letter written on September 20, 1837, to Professor Henslow, in which he reported "an uncomfortable palpitation of the heart." His doctor urged him to rest in the country for a few weeks (10). The palpitations troubled him intermittently for years thereafter.

In a letter to his sister Caroline in May 1838, 18 months after returning to England, the patient wrote: "I find the noodle & the stomach are antagonistic powers, and that it is a great deal more easy to think too much a day than to think too little—what thought has to do with digesting roast beef, I cannot say, but they are brother faculties" (11). This first reference to what he later called "gastric flatus" heralded the onset of a violent abdominal disorder that would plague him for the next three decades.

The patient's gastric disorder consisted of repeated, sudden attacks of abdominal pain, nausea, vomiting, and retching, typically occurring 3 hours after breakfast, and most frequent and severe during times of emotional stress. During the worst periods, which lasted for years on end, he vomited after nearly every meal (12). His bowel movements, however, remained normal (13). Because he seldom regurgitated food, "only acid & morbid secretion" (14), his vomiting did not interfere with his intake or digestion of food, his general nutritional status, or his professional productivity (15). In fact, his scientific output may well have been enhanced under the strictly regulated conditions of the valetudinarian existence his illness forced upon him. In 1974, Sir George Pickering even went so far as to suggest that the patient's illness enabled him to avoid social distractions that would have interfered with his work. "Without the illness," according to Pickering, "the great work would not have been done or done in such a splendid style" (16).

Many of the patient's friends believed he was a hypochondriac (9). His physicians, of whom there were over a score of England's most prominent (17), could find no organic mischief and assured him that eventually he would get over his sickness. His disease was unique, they said, and did not fit any known classification of illness—not quite dyspepsia, nearer to "suppressed gout" (18). Undeterred by their failure to arrive at a definite diagnosis, they prescribed a "non-sugar plan" on the slim possibility that he had a peculiar tendency to oxidize sugar into poisonous oxalic acid, which might benefit by abstaining entirely from sweets (19). Suspecting that he suffered from either "nervous or mucous dyspepsia," Dr. James Gully recommended his own treatment for the former, which consisted of "small feedings of nonirritating food and a hydrotherapy regimen of sitz baths, foot baths, wet sheet packing, and rubbing with a dripping sheet—all of which was supposed to draw blood away from the stomach and produce a counteracting irritation in other organs distant from the stomach" (20).

"Mucous dyspepsia," which was thought to be caused by an underactive, obstructed stomach, was treated by inducing a progressively heightened tolerance to food and exercise along with a hydrotherapy regimen consisting of sweating, followed by a cold shallow bath for 3 or 4 minutes and then a douche and a wet packing. After almost 4 months of such hydrotherapy, the patient believed he had been cured of his gastric flatus and built his own "douche house" outside of his main residence so that he could continue the water treatments at home. Unfortunately, their salutary effect was temporary; eventually, the gastric disorder returned refractory to hydrotherapy (20).

In 1857, after the patient had given up on Gully's water cure, he began taking a mixture of muriatic (hydrochloric) acid and nitric acid for a stomach he had been told was secreting inadequate amounts of acid. This too seemed to relieve his gastric flatus, but only temporarily (21).

Over the course of his three decades of gastric distress the patient's physicians offered a host of additional diagnoses and treatments, none of which succeeded in alleviating his suffering for long. His problem, they claimed was an excess of gastric acid—not insufficient gastric secretion (22), "over-breathing (hyperventilation) (23), an allergic reaction—to medicines, house furnishings, clothing, the vegetation on his grounds, the dogs and cats in his house, etc., etc." (23), and the *Beagle* sickness of September/October 1834 (5).

Not to be outdone by the patient's personal physicians, many would-be diagnosticians since his death have pondered the cause of his invalidism and have added many other diagnoses to the list. These include Chagas disease, neurasthenia, a refractory anomaly of the eyes, mental overwork, schizophrenia, depressive psychosis, chronic appendicitis, a peptic ulcer, chronic cholecystitis, smoldering hepatitis, a diaphragmatic hernia, narcolepsy, hyperinsulinism, arsenicosis, lead poisoning, lactose intolerance, Crohn's disease, panic disorder with agoraphobia, repressed anger toward his father, systemic lupus erythematosus, and cyclic vomiting syndrome (9, 24–27).

The list of treatments administered to the patient in vain during his years of suffering is no less impressive. In addition to those mentioned above, he was treated with small doses of arsenic, calomel, Indian ale, bismuth, Croton (an extract of flowering plants in the spurge family), aloes, lemons, a hydroelectric chain, pepsin, Condy's ozinised water (potassium permanganate solution), magnesium carbonate of ammonia, phosphate of iron, ice therapy, strychnine, and codeine (17).

Whereas the patient's gastric dysfunction was his most distressing complaint, he had many others following his years abroad. These included insomnia, intermittent palpitations (10, 28) and headaches (29), episodes of numbness of the fingertips (30), a buzzing noise in his head (31), stars in his eyes (31), giddiness and trembling hands (in his 30s) (32), and weakness plus a "touch of pleurisy" (at age 51) (33). He had unspecified trouble with his teeth, beginning in his third decade, perhaps related to destruction of tooth enamel by his recurrent vomiting. During his fifth and sixth decades, he wept a great deal while suffering with intermittent "rheumatism/lumbago" (5, 34) and also "boils and eczema" of the face and hands (35, 36). Interestingly, during his fits of rheumatism and eczema his gastric symptoms diminished (37).

The patient's mother died suddenly with abdominal pain when he was 8, of an unknown disorder (38). When she was a child, she was dipped in the icy Irish Sea "to cure her pukes and boils" and as an adult was unable to ride in a carriage without becoming ill. She also had hyperemesis with her pregnancies. Her younger brother, the patient's uncle, suffered with headaches and abdominal pain and was confined to his cabin with seasickness during a voyage to the West Indies taken to improve his health (27).

The patient's father was a prominent physician who lived to the age of 82, though he was morbidly obese and, like his own father and grandfather, suffered with the gout (39). An older brother struggled with depression before dying at age 77 of unknown cause (40). Three sisters died at ages 56, 63, and 88 of unknown causes (40). A paternal great-grandfather and grandmother were alcoholics (41). A paternal half-cousin had digestive problems of unknown character or etiology (42).

The patient's wife, who was also a first cousin, was deeply religious. He desperately wanted to believe what she believed but couldn't accept the Old Testament's revenge-filled deity, and even though trained as a parson at Cambridge, he could never believe what he couldn't understand. His wife worried that his theory, which relied on natural causes rather than on God for the creation of new species, would prevent him from joining her in heaven. Some have speculated that their religious conflict had a role in the origin of the patient's invalidism (43).

They had 10 children (7 sons and 3 daughters) (44). Three died young. Five developed hypochondriacal concerns about their health, possibly prompted by their father's expressed conviction that his own disorder was hereditary (45); four of the children had fluctuating digestive troubles less severe than their father's (44); and several exhibited a "tendency for irregular pulses," possibly induced by the repeated examinations to which they were subjected by their father (46).

The patient was tall (6′) and lean as a youth, with a light complexion and reddish-brown hair that receded rapidly after puberty. By all accounts he was a modest, humble, and eminently likeable man, who was all eyes. "Nothing escaped him. No object in nature, whether flower or bird or insect of any kind, could avoid his loving recognition. He knew them all" (47). Though possessed of steely intellectual courage, he "dearly loved a joke, laughing with a mock-mischievous expression that took you captive" (47).

He was addicted to snuff (48), which he used several times a day from age 18. He drank brandy, wine, and port in moderation (49). Walking was his only exercise (50).

During his final decade, the patient's physical health improved markedly, with absence of "serious exacerbations of vomiting" (51, 52). However, by his seventh decade, his memory was beginning to fail (53). He began to complain of constant attacks of "swimming of the head" (54) and "some pain in the heart" (55). While rock climbing at the age of 72, he experienced a sudden "fit of dazzling" (56). The precise character of the fit is uncertain but likely involved "giddiness and an irregular pulse," in that he reported these 3 months later. He then developed a cough, which quinine seemed to alleviate (57). Shortly thereafter he experienced precordial (anterior chest) pain, giddiness, exhaustion, and insomnia. Amyl nitrate provided little relief. Sitting at dinner one evening, he was seized with giddiness and fainted while trying to reach a sofa. Within minutes he regained consciousness, drank some brandy, and seemed to recover. He then became nauseated and began vomiting and retching violently. This lasted until the next day, April 19, 1882, when he again lost consciousness and died. He was 73 years and 2 months old. The cause of death was listed as "angina attacks with heart failure and degeneration of the heart and greater blood vessels" (58).

Charles Darwin (Fig. 10.1) had intended to be buried in a rough-hewn wooden coffin beside his brother. The Royal Society, the Dean of Westminster, and the British Parliament, however, would not hear of a man who had brought so much honor to the English name lying in an obscure grave. And so, on April 26, 1882, his remains were placed in a casket so highly polished "you could see your face in it," transported to Westminster Abbey, and buried with all the pomp and ceremony worthy of as great a man of science as ever searched for truth (59).

Of the myriad diagnoses offered over the years to explain Darwin's long suffering, given the nature of his complaints, only three merit serious consideration—cyclic vomiting syndrome, hypochondriasis, and Chagas disease.

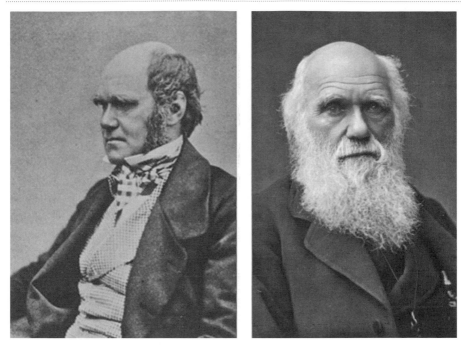

FIGURE 10.1 Charles Darwin ca. 1854 at age 45 (*left*) and ca. 1881 at age 72 (*right*).

Cyclic vomiting syndrome (60, 61) is a little-known yet surprisingly common and disabling disorder characterized by recurrent episodes of nausea, vomiting, and abdominal pain separated by asymptomatic intervals. Migraine headaches are common, in patients as well as their family members, as are cardiac arrhythmias and other manifestations of dysautonomia (as, for example, Darwin's numbness of his fingertips and nervous tics). The intense anxiety precipitated by uncontrollable episodes of vomiting occasionally induces behavior mimicking an affective or anxiety disorder—two of the many psychiatric disorders attributed to Darwin—or an endocrine disorder such as hypothyroidism or hypoglycemia.

Cyclic vomiting syndrome is, in essence, a diagnosis of exclusion, in which standard diagnostic tests for recurrent vomiting are uniformly negative. Many patients, however, exhibit evidence of defective mitochondria—tiny organelles present within all mammalian cells, except red blood cells, that produce much of the energy supporting normal cellular function (62). At least some patients with cyclic vomiting syndrome possess a mutation of a particular mitochondrial gene known as A3243G. Considerable evidence supports a matrilineal pattern of inheritance of the disorder, in which case Darwin likely inherited it from his mother, a member of the Wedgwood family, and his children from their mother, also a Wedgwood.

Although commonly presenting during the preschool to early school-age years, cyclic vomiting syndrome can begin at any time from infancy to adulthood, with reported ages of onset ranging from 2 to 49 years. Darwin's episodes of vomiting began in his teens, when he had an upset stomach mainly after breakfast. In adult patients, episodes are typically stereotypical (i.e., similar in duration and character one episode to the next) over months to years, with attacks most often arising between midnight and noon. In men, vomiting is commonly triggered by noxious stress, pleasant excitement, and/or infections, whereas in women, triggers include menstruation, noxious stress, pleasant excitement, and/or fatigue. In Darwin's case, episodes of vomiting were frequently triggered by noxious stress and pleasant excitement but were alleviated by his skin eruptions.

The differential diagnosis for cyclic vomiting syndrome is broad (Table 10.1). In addition to the alternative diagnoses mentioned above, many others are pursued in the diagnostic evaluation of these patients. In the state of Maryland today, to take one typical example, the Hospital Services Cost Review Commission (HSCRC)/ Medicare-approved charges for the studies listed in Table 10.1 total $11,220 if performed only once, not including professional fees paid to a primary care provider or subspecialty consultants, or charges associated with emergency room visits or hospitalizations (63).

In many adult patients, prolonged showers or baths lessen the intensity of attacks; however, in contrast to Darwin's hydrotherapy, which afforded him temporary relief, most current patients report benefit from exposure to hot rather than cold water. Although no experimentally validated treatment for the disorder has proved to be effective, many are prescribed in an effort to relieve the suffering of these patients. These treatments include intravenous hydration, antimigraine drugs, such as amitriptyline, propranolol, and cyproheptadine, anxiolytics/ antiemetics, such as ondansetron, lorazepam, and alprazolam, analgesics, such as ibuprofen and oxycodone, and antacids, such as H2 blockers and proton-pump inhibitors. Emergency room visits are frequent, hospital admissions less so. Many patients undergo cholecystectomies to no avail; a few are subjected needlessly to other abdominal surgical procedures, such as appendectomy, exploratory laparotomy, pyloroplasty, gastrostomy and jejunostomy, and fundoplication.

One can only guess how many of these tests and treatments Darwin would receive if he were a patient today. Given the severity of his gastric disorder and his obsession with it, it is likely that he would be subjected to most, if not all. Although his episodes of vomiting lasted substantially longer than those experienced by patients meeting the current definition for the syndrome (the Rome III diagnostic criteria (64)), the preponderance of evidence contained in his medical history is more consistent with the syndrome than any other diagnosis yet proposed for his "gastric flatus." If this, in fact, were his problem, none of the tests and treatments listed above would either diagnose or cure his ailment.

TABLE 10.1

Diagnostic Evaluation of Patients with Cyclic Vomiting Syndrome (60, 61)

Alternative Diagnosis[1]	Diagnostic Tests	Potential Harm Caused by the Tests
Esophageal reflux[a]	EGD, UGI, PPI trial	Bleeding, cardiopulmonary complications of sedation, bowel perforation, aspiration
Gastritis/PUD/ achalasia[a]	EGD (with biopsy), antibody assay and/or stool antigen or breath test for *H. pylori*	Bleeding, cardiopulmonary complications of sedation, bowel perforation, aspiration
Pancreatitis[a]	Serum amylase and lipase, endoscopic ultrasound	Bleeding, cardiopulmonary complications of sedation, bowel perforation, aspiration
Gallbladder disease[a,b]	Abdominal ultrasound, endoscopic retrograde cholangio-pancreatography	Bleeding, cardiopulmonary complications of sedation, bowel perforation, aspiration, pancreatitis
Partial bowel obstruction[a,b]	UGI (with small bowel follow-through), colonoscopy, abdominal CT scan (with contrast)	Bowel perforation, bleeding, radiation exposure, contrast-induced ARF
Pyelonephritis	Urinalysis, urine culture and sensitivity	None
Appendicitis[a,b]	CBC, abdominal CT scan (with contrast)	Radiation exposure, contrast-induced ARF
Delayed gastric emptying[a]	Radionucleotide gastric emptying study	Radiation exposure
Porphyria[c]	Urine porphyrins	None
Plumbism	Whole blood lead concentration	None
Abdominal epilepsy/ migraine[d]	EEG, head CT (with contrast) and MRI (with gadolinium), antimigraine drug trial	Radiation exposure, contrast-induced ARF, gadolinium-induce nephrogenic sclerosis
Crohn's disease[a]	EGD, abdominal CT (with contrast), colonoscopy, capsule endoscopy	Bleeding, bowel perforation, radiation exposure

(*continued*)

TABLE 10.1 (*Continued*)

Alternative Diagnosis[1]	Diagnostic Tests	Potential Harm Caused by the Tests
SLE[e]	Assays for antinuclear, anti-double-stranded DNA and anti-Sm nuclear antigen antibodies	None
Psychiatric disorder[d,f]	EEG, head CT (with contrast) and MRI/MRA (with gadolinium)	Radiation exposure, contrast-induced ARF, gadolinium-induced nephrogenic sclerosis
Chagas disease[g]	*T. cruzi* antibody assay	None

[1]*Subspecialty consultation obtained*: a, Gastroenterology; b, General surgery; c, Endocrinology; d, Neurology; e, Rheumatology; f, Psychiatry; g, Infectious diseases.

PUD, peptic ulcer disease; SLE, systemic lupus erythematosus; EGD, esophagogastric duodenoscopy; UGI, upper gastrointestinal barium study; PPI, proton pump inhibitor; CBC, complete blood count; CT, computed tomography; MRI, magnetic resonance imaging; MRA, magnetic resonance angiography; EEG, electroencephalogram; ARF, acute renal failure.

Hypochondriasis (65) is classified under the somatization disorders in the American Psychiatric Association's *Diagnostic and Statistical Manual of Mental Disorders, Fourth Edition* (DSM-IV (66)). It is characterized by an obsessive irrational fear of having a serious medical condition despite the failure of a comprehensive medical evaluation to identify any such condition. Although the belief is not of delusional intensity, attempts at reassurance fail to alleviate the patient's fear.

Table 10.2 lists the DSM-IV criteria defining hypochondriasis, many of which are fulfilled by Darwin's illness. For three decades he was certainly preoccupied with fears of a serious disease despite repeatedly negative medical evaluations and reassurance from numerous physicians that he had no such disease. He was not delusional or obsessively concerned about his appearance. His gastric disorder was a source of considerable distress. It did not, however, impair his social or occupational effectiveness to any significant degree. Of the alternative diagnoses listed in Table 10.2, only panic disorder has more than a few features typical of Darwin's illness. Panic disorder has been reported to coexist with hypochondriasis in 10 to 20 percent of cases.

Unlike Darwin, patients suffering with hypochondriasis typically are reluctant to acknowledge the role of psychological factors in causing their symptoms; misinterpret benign physical sensations as evidence of serious illness; tend to respond to reassurance with anger rather than relief; and frequently are functionally impaired to a severe degree by the disorder. Darwin, in fact, recognized the role of

TABLE 10.2

DSM-IV Diagnostic Criteria for 300.7, Hypochondriasis (66)

A. Preoccupation with fears of having, or the idea that one has, a serious disease based on the person's misinterpretation of bodily symptoms.

B. The preoccupation persists despite appropriate medical evaluation and reassurance.

C. The belief in Criterion A is not of delusional intensity (as in Delusional Disorder, Somatic Type) and is not restricted to a circumscribed concern about appearance (as in Body Dysmorphic Disorder).

D. The preoccupation causes clinically significant distress or impairment in social, occupational, or other important areas of functioning.

E. The duration of the disturbance is at least 6 months.

F. The preoccupation is not better accounted for by Generalized Anxiety Disorder, Obsessive-Compulsive Disorder, Panic Disorder, a Major Depressive Episode, Separation Anxiety, or another Somatoform Disorder.

anxiety caused by his revolutionary concepts in precipitating his gastric distress; had physical sensations that were hardly "benign"; was a compliant and grateful patient; and in spite of his symptoms, continued to function effectively as husband, father, friend, colleague, and scientist.

Like patients with cyclic vomiting syndrome, those with hypochondriasis have high rates of visits to physicians, subspecialty consultations, laboratory tests, and surgical procedures, all of which lead to high health care costs. Despite such intense medical attention, their symptoms generally remain unabated. Although cognitive, pharmacological, and several other therapies have been recommended for the disorder, proof of clinical efficacy has yet to be demonstrated for any of these treatments.

In October 1959, Professor Saul Adler (9), a world-renowned parasitologist, proposed Chagas disease (67) as the cause of Darwin's prolonged gastric distress, citing a previously unnoticed passage from the *Beagle* narrative in which Darwin described being bitten by "the great black bug of the Pampas," the principal vector for this infection. For years Adler's theory dominated thinking as to the etiology of Darwin's "gastric flatus," but it has since fallen into disfavor (68). If the gastric symptoms Darwin experienced as a teenager were the initial manifestations of his "gastric flatus," as seems likely, Chagas disease could not have been the cause, since his exposure to the infection would only have occurred after the onset of the illness. Therefore, if he suffered with Chagas disease, the infection would have been in the form of a cardiomyopathy rather than one of the digestive "mega" syndromes (Chagas-induced enlargement of the esophagus and/or colon) as originally proposed. Chagas disease might explain his terminal cardiac symptoms and perhaps amplified his gastric disorder indirectly by facilitating invasion of his stomach by *Helicobacter pylori* (see below).

Chagas disease is caused by the protozoan parasite *Trypanosoma cruzi* (67). The microbe is transmitted to humans and many other animals mainly by great black, bloodsucking bugs belonging to the subfamily Triatominae, of which only a small number are competent vectors.

In March 1835, Darwin was bitten by one such bug (a great black Benchuca bug) while residing in the Pampas of Argentina. More than likely he was bitten repeatedly by such bugs during his excursions in both Argentina and Chile, and might well have been infected by *T. cruzi* in the process.

Recent surveys, however, have indicated that only a small percentage of people at risk of *T. cruzi* infection (i.e., those exposed to Benchucas harboring the parasite) are actually infected (17.4 percent), and of those infected, less than half develop clinically apparent disease. The acute phase of symptomatic infections lasts 4 to 6 weeks and is characterized by prolonged fever, malaise, hepatosplenomegaly, lymphadenopathy, and occasionally cardiac arrhythmias (67).

The chronic phase of the disease usually does not manifest clinically until 10 to 30 years after the initial infection. The digestive form, which develops in only 10 to 15 percent of chronically infected patients, consists of mega-esophagus, mega-colon, or both. Darwin never exhibited signs or symptoms of either. The cardiac form of the disease, the most serious and frequent manifestation of chronic Chagas disease, develops in 20 to 30 percent of chronically infected patients. It typically produces abnormalities of the cardiac conduction system as well as bradyarrhythmias (slow pulse), tachyarrhythmias (rapid pulse), apical aneurysms, heart failure, thromboembolism, and sudden death (67). Thus, Chagas cardiomyopathy might have been the cause of Darwin's terminal cardiac dysfunction and death. However, given his age at the time his heart began to fail, his failing memory, and the infrequency with which persons exposed to Benchuca bugs develop the chronic form of the disease, it is more likely that he died of atherosclerosis of the arteries of his heart and brain. In the chronic phase, Chagas disease is diagnosed by demonstrating the presence of antibodies against *T. cruzi*. If alive today, Darwin would certainly be tested for these and more than likely would also have his cardiac and cerebral symptoms extensively evaluated with an electrocardiogram (EKG), Holter monitor, stress test, and cardiac catheterization, along with a computed tomographic scan and magnetic resonance imaging of his head.

Although the drugs benznidazole and nifurtimox are effective against acute Chagas disease, they are not recommended for patients with advanced cardiac disease. Cardiac symptoms are managed with the drug amiodarone, a cardiac pace-maker and implantable defibrillator, along with diuretics and beta-blockers, even though the efficacy of this combination of therapies has not been confirmed in clinical trials (67). Today, Darwin would no doubt be given many, if not most, of these in managing his cardiac symptoms.

For reasons yet to be determined, patients with Chagas disease are prone to infection with the bacterium *H. pylori* (69), which in its acute phase causes vomiting, abdominal pain, and weight loss. During the chronic phase of such infections, a small minority of patients develop gastritis, peptic ulcer disease, gastric cancer, or lymphoma. Dr. Barry Marshall, the co-discoverer of *H. pylori*'s role in peptic ulcer disease, believes that Darwin's gastric distress was caused by the bacterium (70). If so, Darwin's particular disorder more likely would have been a peculiarly persistent form of *H. pylori*-induced chronic gastritis (i.e., non-ulcer dyspepsia) than a peptic ulcer, gastric cancer, or lymphoma. Unfortunately, current treatments have little if any effect on the course of such dyspepsia (71).

According to a descendent of the great man, in Darwin's home "it was a distinction and a mournful pleasure to be ill" (72). Darwin might have been a hypochondriac, as implied by this statement, and today would be seen by a psychiatrist in consultation and also subjected to psychological testing. However, for the reasons given above, cyclic vomiting syndrome is a more likely diagnosis, as is atherosclerotic cardiovascular disease as the cause of his death. Although his physicians, some of the finest Britain had to offer at the time, could find no physical abnormality to explain his gastric symptoms, they had only Darwin's history and physical examination to guide them in their evaluations.

When Darwin was the subject of a historical clinicopathological conference at the University of Maryland School of Medicine in 2011, Mr. Wayne Millan, for many years a co-organizer of the conference, gave a brief monologue in which he imagined Darwin's father's reaction to the conclusions summarized above. Dr. Robert Darwin, he speculated, would have offered his modern counterparts the following advice based on comments contained in letters the doctor wrote to his son: "The sure knowledge that we all have a measured portion of life—some of us long, many of us short—our aim must be to further the quality of that life rather than to imagine we can alter it so fundamentally as to live forever." Darwin's physicians' many treatments did little to further either the quality or the length of his life. Could present-day physicians have done more?

If Darwin were alive today, no doubt a wide array of sophisticated laboratory examinations would be added to his workup. Those directed at his "gastric flatus" more than likely would be uniformly negative. Nevertheless, a modern-day clinician, driven by both the patient's expectations and those of third-party payers, would not likely abandon Darwin without presenting him with a diagnosis and instituting his or her own welter of treatments. Physicians specializing in disorders of the upper gastrointestinal tract most likely would diagnose cyclic vomiting syndrome after all other diagnoses had been excluded through a comprehensive battery of negative tests. This "diagnosis of exclusion" would be offered to Darwin as reassurance that his illness was not imaginary and that he was not alone in his suffering. It would not, however, provide insight into the disorder's cause, the mechanisms by which it arose or was sustained, or an effective means of preventing or curing it. Like diagnoses such as irritable bowel syndrome, attention-deficit disorder, chronic hyperventilation syndrome, restless leg syndrome, sudden infant death syndrome, posttraumatic stress disorder, and many others given to patients today, "cyclic vomiting syndrome" does little more than paraphrase the complaints for which the patient seeks medical attention. Ultimately, it is no more enlightening or helpful in relieving the suffering of patients like Darwin than "excess gastric acid" or "suppressed gout" or "mucous dyspepsia" was over a century ago (63).

The modern diagnostic studies directed at Darwin's terminal cardiac dysfunction almost certainly would reveal advanced atherosclerosis of the arteries of both his heart and brain. Here again, although a host of treatments would be given for the disorder, it is not likely that any would prove more than marginally better in relieving Darwin's suffering or extending his life than those administered by his own physicians so many years ago. Thus, the best that can be said of the capacity of modern medicine to relieve the suffering of patients like Darwin is that:

Not to go back is somewhat to advance
And men must walk, at least, before they dance. (73)◆

References

1. Huxley TH. Obituary notices of fellows deceased. *Proc Roy Soc* 1888;44:i–xxv.

2. Evans JP. The voyage continues. Darwin and medicine at 200 years. *JAMA* 2009;301:663–665.

3. Colp R, Jr. *To Be an Invalid. The illness of Charles Darwin.* Chicago: The University of Chicago Press, 1977:17.

4. Barlow N, ed. *The Autobiography of Charles Darwin, 1809–1882* (with original omissions restored). London: Collins, 1958:68.

5. Op. cit. Colp, p. 113.

6. Barlow N, ed. *Charles Darwin's Diary of the Voyage of H.M.S. "Beagle."* Cambridge: Cambridge University Press, 1833:42, 61.

7. Barlow N, ed. *Charles Darwin and the Voyage of the "Beagle."* New York: Philosophical Library, 1946:160.

8. Op. cit. Colp, pp. 10–11.

9. Adler S. Darwin's illness. *Nature* 1959;184:1102–1103.

10. Barlow N, ed. *Darwin and Henslow: The Growth of an Idea*. London: John Murray, 1967:136.

11. Charles Darwin Papers and letters (DPL). *Handlist of Darwin Papers of the University Library*. Cambridge: Cambridge University Press, 1960, Darwin to Mrs. Caroline Wedgwood, May 1838.

12. Darwin Correspondence Project (DCP) (www.darwinproject.ac.uk), Darwin to Hooker, March 31, 1845 (letter 847).

13. Op. cit. Colp, p. 22.

14. Op. cit. DCP, Darwin to Hooker, February 22, 1864 (letter 4412).

15. Op. cit. Colp, pp. 15–85.

16. Ibid., p. 105.

17. Ibid., pp. 279–80.

18. Ibid., p. 39.

19. Ibid., p. 37.

20. Ibid., pp. 40–43.

21. Ibid., p. 57.

22. Ibid., p. 78.

23. Ibid., p. 98.

24. Young DAB. Darwin's illness and systemic lupus erythematosus. *Notes Records Roy Soc London* 1997;51:77–86.

25. Barloon TJ, Noyes R, Jr. Charles Darwin and panic disorder. *JAMA* 1997;277:138–41.

26. Orrego F, Quintana C. Darwin's illness: a final diagnosis. *Notes Records Roy Soc* 2007;61:23–29.

27. Hayman JA. Darwin's illness revisited. *BMJ* 2009;339:1413–1415.

28. Op. cit. DCP, Darwin to Hooker, December 4, 1860 (letter 3008).

29. De Beer G, ed. Darwin's journal. *Bull Brit Museum* (*Natural History*) 1959; Historical Series 2:1–21.

30. Litchfield H, ed. *Emma Darwin: A Century of Family Letters, 1792–1896*. London: John Murray, 1915: vol. 2, p. 87.

31. Hooker J. Reminiscences of Darwin. *Nature* 1899;60:188

32. Op. cit. DCP, Darwin to Hooker, March 28, 1849 (letter 1236).

33. Ibid., Darwin to Asa Gray, March 2, 1860 (letter 2718).

34. Op. cit. Colp, p. 136.

35. Op. cit. DCP, Darwin to Hooker, June 23, 1862 (letter 3620).

36. Ibid., Darwin to Hooker, June 30, 1862 (letter 3628).

37. Ibid., Darwin to Hooker, February 9, 1865 (letter 4769).

38. Op. cit. Colp, p. 246.

39. King-Hele D. *Erasmus Darwin*. New York: Charles Scribner's Sons, 1963:14, 32–33.

40. Op. cit. Colp, p. 119.

41. Op. cit. Autobiography, p. 224.

42. Litchfield RB. *Tom Wedgwood: the First Photographer*. London: Duckworth & Co., 1903:23–24.

43. Op. cit. Autobiography, p. 237.

44. Op. cit. Colp, pp. 45, 63, 69, 120–121.

45. Op. cit. DCP, Darwin to Fox, March 7, 1852 (letter 1476).

46. Ibid., Darwin to Hooker, October 6, 1858 (letter 2335).

47. Op. cit. Colp, p. 60.

48. Op. cit. DCP, Darwin to Fox, March 24, 1849 (letter 1235).

49. Ibid., Darwin to Hooker, October 4, 1863 (letter 4318).

50. Op. cit. Colp, p. 34.

51. Op. cit. DPL, Henrietta Litchfield to Francis Darwin, March 18, 1887.

52. Nash LA. Some memories of Charles Darwin. *Overland Monthly* 1921;771:27.

53. Op. cit. DCP, Darwin to Hooker, September 12, 1873 (letter 9052).

54. Ibid., Darwin to Hooker, March 2, 1878 (letter 11390).

55. Atkins H. *Down. The Home of the Darwins. The Story of a House and the People Who Lived There*. London: Royal College of Surgeons, 1974:38.

56. Op. cit. Litchfield, vol. 2, p. 247.

57. Darwin F, Seward AC, eds. *More Letters of Charles Darwin. A Record of his Work in a Series of Hitherto Unpublished Letters*. New York: Appleton & Co., 1903, vol. 2, pp. 446–447.

58. Op. cit. Colp, pp. 94–96.

59. Padel R. *Darwin. A Life in Poems*. New York: Alfred A. Knopf, 2009:140.

60. Fleisher DR, Gornowicz B, Adams K, Burch R, Feldman EJ. Cyclic vomiting syndrome in 41 adults: the illness, the patients, and problems of management. *BMC Med* 2005;3:20–32.

61. Boles RG, Adams K, Li BUK. Maternal inheritance in cyclic vomiting syndrome. *Am J Med Genetics* 2005;133A:71–77.

62. Wallace DC. A mitochondrial paradigm of metabolic and degenerative diseases, aging and cancer: a dawn for evolutionary medicine. *Ann Rev Genet* 2005;39:359–407.

63. Cohen S, Mackowiak PA. Diagnosing Darwin. *The Pharos*, Spring 2013:14–20).

64. Tack J, Talley NJ. Gastroduodenal disorders. *Am J Gastroenterol* 2010;105:757–763.

65. Barsky AJ. The patient with hypochondriasis. *N Engl J Med* 2001;345:1395–1399.

66. American Psychiatric Association. *Diagnostic and Statistical Manual of Mental Disorders*, 4th ed. (DSM IV). Washington, DC: American Psychiatric Association, 2000.

67. Rassi A, Jr, Rassi A, Marin-Neto JA. Chagas disease. *Lancet* 2010;375:1388–1402.

68. Woodruff AW. Darwin's health in relation to his voyage to South America. *BMJ* 1965;1:745–750.

69. Matsuda NM, Miller SM, Evora PRB. The chronic gastrointestinal manifestations of Chagas disease. *Clinics (Sao Paulo)* 2009;64:1219–1224.

70. Marshall B. *Darwin's illness was Helicobacter pylori*. WHAT I KNOW AND WHAT I THINK I KNOW. (blog), posted Feb. 13, 2009.

71. Blaser MF. *Helicobacter pylori* and other gastric Helicobacter species. In Mandell GL, Bennett JE, Dolin R, eds. *Principles and Practice of Infectious Diseases*, 7th ed. Philadelphia: Churchill, Livingstone Elsevier, 2010:2803–2813.

72. Sharp D. Forebears and heirs; a sketch. *Lancet* 2008 (Darwin's Gifts supplement) S40–S43.

73. Pope A. *Imitations of Horace*. I, I, l. 53.

The revolutionary despises all doctrines and refuses to accept the mundane sciences, leaving them for future generations. He knows only one science: the science of destruction.

SERGEY GENNADIYEVICH NECHAYEV, The Revolutionary Catechism (1)

11 Vessels of Stone

TROTSKY, GORKY, DAN, MARTOV, ZINOVIEV, AND STALIN were this patient's acolytes. For years he conspired with them against the Romanovs, mostly while in exile, before returning to Russia aboard a famous "sealed train"—repatriated during the First World War by the German General Staff in the hope that he would weaken the Russian war effort. When the patient arrived at St. Petersburg's Finland Station in April 1917, he mounted an armored car and, in the glare of searchlights, proclaimed the beginning of the worldwide socialist revolution. Within a few months he was ruler of Russia; in another 7 years he was dead (2).

Prior revolutions had limited themselves to the overthrow of one political system to replace it with another. His revolution was different—one Nechayev would have applauded (3). It destroyed the entire state to its roots and exterminated all the state traditions, institutions, and classes. It reduced the infinite variety of social and intellectual life, culture, historical tradition, and the creative potential of millions of people to a harsh, uniform, uncompromising ideological paradigm (4).

The patient was a theorist and a rhetorician of revolution more than a leader (5). He never handled bombs, kettles, or acid himself (6), nor did he have any inclination to kill or to maim personally or even to witness butchery. However, he took cruel delight in recommending merciless terror (6). For him, no moral threshold was sacred. He rejected concepts of conscience, compassion, and charity (7), introduced the term "enemy of the people," urged the taking of hostages, and created penal units and concentration camps. He called for "shooting on the spot" and made informing on one's neighbors a patriotic duty (8). He banned the non-Bolshevik press, expelled the Russian intelligentsia, destroyed provincial administrations, squandered the country's wealth on a world revolution, and created crime-urging hunger throughout Mother Russia that left millions dead of starvation. All this he did without remorse, in the firm belief that the end always justifies the means (9).

The Bolsheviks laid the foundation for his unique state in the year and a half following the October Revolution. The State had a single ruling party to which the legislature, executive, and judiciary were all subordinate. The Party was the supreme state agency, and he was its supreme leader (10). Without him, there would have been no October Revolution in 1917. Without him, the Russian Communist Party would not have survived beyond the end of 1921 (11), and a third of the inhabited world would not have been ruled by communist regimes for decades after the Second World War (10).

He died in 1924, a few months shy of his 54th birthday, with cerebral vessels so calcified that when tapped with tweezers, they sounded like stone (12). His crimes against humanity during his brief life were monstrous. And yet, when surveys of Russian opinion are taken today, he remains among the most popular rulers in history (13).

He was born in Simbirsk, Russia, on April 23, 1870 (14). He was a mischievous child, with short, weak legs and a head so large he was top-heavy and had trouble maintaining his balance. He learned to walk late and had an odd habit of crashing his head on the floor when he didn't get his way. His mother wondered if he might be mentally retarded (15). However, although he never lost his impulsive and choleric temperament, as he grew into manhood, his mother and the world came to realize that he was endowed with extraordinary intellectual vitality (16).

He suffered greatly with insomnia, migraines, and abdominal pain during his adult years, especially when under stress (17). He had "a mild bout of typhoid" at age 22 (18), intermittent toothaches (19), and an attack of erysipelas when he was 33 (20). Twice he was knocked off his bicycle and badly bruised—once when 34 and again at age 38 (21). He contracted influenza at age 37 (22). A year later, he was shot during one of several assassination attempts. A bullet pierced his left scapula, punctured his lung, and came to rest near his right clavicle. A second bullet lodged in the base of his neck. He was treated conservatively and recovered (23, 24).

He had seven siblings, two of whom died as infants. An older brother was executed when he was 21 for conspiring to assassinate Tsar Alexander III. An older sister had a stroke at age 71 and died. Two younger sisters and a younger brother succumbed, respectively, to typhoid fever (age 19), a heart attack (age 59), and "stenocardia" (angina) (age 69) (25). His brother Sasha and his sister Anna suffered with headaches, insomnia, and abdominal pains similar to his (17).

The patient's antecedents were Russian, Kalmyk, Jewish, German, and Swedish (26). His maternal grandfather was a doctor and a Jew who renounced his religious heritage (27). His father was an inspector and, later, a provincial director of schools. He died at age 54, following a period of mental decline similar to that experienced by the patient (28). Although the father was given a diagnosis of cerebral hemorrhage, his symptoms at the time of his death (persistent cough and rigors) were more consistent with pneumonia (29). The patient's mother died at age 81 of unknown cause (30). The family was well off financially and intellectually gifted.

The patient trained as a lawyer but spent little time in the practice of law (31). Though married at age 28, he had no children (32). Affairs of the heart never got in the way of his political activities (33). However, he did have a mistress. She was an advocate of free love, whom he met when he was 40 (34). She developed tuberculosis 2 years after meeting him and in another 8 years died of cholera (35).

The patient didn't smoke and prohibited smoking in his presence (36). He drank alcohol sparingly and, except for a fondness for mushrooms (37), took little interest in the quality of his food other than to avoid oily foods, which tended to upset his stomach (38). He exercised regularly, swimming, biking, walking, and/or hunting as often as his hectic schedule allowed (39, 40).

His temperament was that of "a pressure-cooker on the stove waiting to blow its lid" (5). Everything about him reflected impatience and determination (41). He became visibly agitated and pale under stress, did everything "in a panic…everything angrily" (42). Only when fishing did he relax (15). He was obsessively tidy (43) and intolerant of extraneous noise (44, 45). When he was 30, he began consulting specialists in nervous disorders for his bad nerves (45).

Before the patient's party came to power, he enjoyed a free and easy existence, unburdened by routine. Afterward, he worked with a driving urgency, hardly bothering to undress before falling into an exhausted, troubled sleep. After the revolution, brief naps no longer refreshed him. Every day he wrote articles and gave speeches in countless venues while contending with some new disaster. Every day he woke with a dull headache (46).

The demands of state service forced him to shift his attention from economic to political questions, from Party to diplomatic concerns, and to deal with endless streams of visitors. The transition from émigré spectator of Russian public life and its sternest critic to the epicenter of upheavals caused by his policies overloaded a nervous system that had never been particularly strong. Tense events and new dangers caused him to erupt in anger and to turn pale. The sound of a violin put his nerves on edge, as did almost any extraneous noise. When his apartment in the Kremlin was remodeled, he ordered partitions between rooms to be made absolutely soundproof and the floors completely free of squeaks. If people talked out of turn during his meetings, he became enraged (45).

In time, his nerves became so frayed that he could barely work. As his stress increased, so did his bellicosity and his barbarism. In a state of heightened excitement during the fight against the Cossacks in 1905, he fulminated for the use of "knives, knuckle-busters, sticks, paraffin-soaked rags, nails, slabs of gun-cotton, boiling water, stones and acid to throw over the police." When his nervous instability intensified after his first major stroke, psychiatrists and neurologists were consulted. They concluded that the basis of his illness was "overstrain of the brain" complicated by "a severe disorder of [its] blood vessels" (45).

Except for the sly, shifty eyes of a wolf (47), there was little physically to suggest the existence of the patient's inner turmoil or his towering intellect. He was short with broad shoulders and large, ugly hands. He had a pleasant, swarthy, slightly Asiatic face, with piercing, dark brown eyes, left strabismus, and a broad forehead and high cheekbones. He had a hoarse voice, a bloated physique, and haggard features that made him seem older than he was (30). As a youth he had had fiery red hair, but by the time he reached his early 20s, he was nearly completely bald (28, 30).

He literally "fizzed with intellectual vitality" (16). In school he, like his siblings, was nearly always at the top of his class (48). He played chess at the level of a master (49). And when he was prevented from studying law at a Russian imperial university, he registered as an external student at St. Petersburg University to prepare for the jurisprudence exams (50). His capacity for assimilating information quickly was such that when he took the exams a year later, he received the highest possible grade in every subject, the only student in his year to do so (31).

The patient's health began a sudden, sharp decline in mid-1921 when he was 51 and could no longer work at his usual frenetic pace because of worsening headaches, insomnia, and "a series of small heart attacks" (51). In November of that year, while addressing the Fourth Congress of the Communist Party in German (one of three languages in which he was fluent), he had difficulty finding words and began snapping his fingers, trying to bring them to mind. He had his first major stroke in May of the next year, in response to which a Central Committee plenum passed a special resolution placing Stalin in charge of his medical care (52). He was seen by some of Europe's most prominent physicians for these complaints. Initially, they thought he was suffering from mental exhaustion (53), possibly neurasthenia (54). Later, when his neurological problems progressed, they wondered if lead leaking from the bullet lodged in his neck was the source of his neurological disorder and removed it (55). Eventually, they treated him for syphilis with injections of an arsenic-based preparation in spite of several alleged negative Wasserman tests (blood tests for syphilis), the official reports of which have since vanished (56). He had another

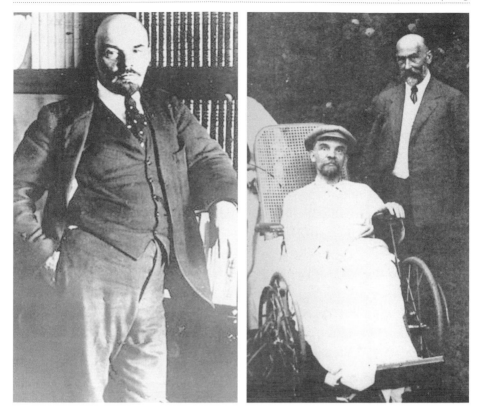

FIGURE 11.1 Lenin at the height of his power (*left*) and at Gorki in July–August 1923 (*right*), showing evidence of the striking deterioration in his condition that evolved during the 2 years before he died. The man standing beside him is unidentified, possibly a physician.

major stroke 6 months after the first and then a third 3 months after that. On January 21, 1924, Vladimir Ilich Ulyanov (Lenin, a.k.a. Peterburzhets, Starik, Ilyin, Frei, Petrov, Maier, Iordanov, Richter, Karpov, Mueller, and Tulin (57)) (Fig. 11.1) died following a series of "convulsions that hurled his small body from one side of the bed to the other" (58). He was 3 months shy of his 54th birthday.

An autopsy was performed the next day (59). The principal findings were as follows:

> ...In the left clavicle at the border of the lower and middle third there is a slight thickening of the bone. Above this area in the posterior part of the deltoid...a deformed bullet is found...enclosed in a capsule of connective tissue...Upon removing the skull cover, a solid fusion of the dura mater with the inner surface of the cranium is noted, primarily along the course of the longitudinal sinus...The anterior part of the left hemisphere seems slightly collapsed in comparison with the corresponding part of the right hemisphere...Brain. Weight immediately

after removal, freed of the dura mater, is 1,340 g. In the left hemisphere...there are noticeable signs of pronounced collapse of the cerebral surface. In the right hemisphere at the border between the temporal and occipital poles there are also two adjacent spots of collapse of the brain surface...In some areas...the arachnoid is hard and appears thickened upon section...Both arteriae vertibralis, and also the arteria basilaris are thickened, do not collapse; their walls are hard, irregularly thickened, of a whitish and in places yellowish color. Upon section, their lumen is seen to be extremely narrowed in places down to the dimensions of a tiny slit. Identical changes are also found in branches of the arteries in question (aa. Cerebri posteriors). The internal carotid arteries, and also the anterior cerebral arteries are similarly hardened, with an irregularly thickened wall and in spots greatly narrowed lumen. The left internal carotid artery in its intracranial course has a completely obliterated lumen and upon section appears merely as a homogeneous solid whitish band. The left Sylvian [i.e., middle cerebral] artery is very thin, hardened, but upon section still shows a thin small slit...In the above noted areas of collapse of the brain there are areas of softening of the tissue, having a yellowish color and accompanied by formation of cyst-like structures filled with a turbid liquid...the corpora quadrigemina...there are signs of fresh hemorrhage in this area...The omentum and the mesentery are rich in fat...The interior of the ascending aorta shows a small number of convex yellowish plaques. The wall thickness of the left ventricle is 1¾ cm and of the right 1 cm. The coronary arteries gape upon section; their walls are very hard and thickened; their lumen definitely constricted. The inner surface of the descending aorta and also the inner surfaces of the large arteries in general show numerous very prominent yellowish plaques, partly undergoing ulceration and calcification...The kidneys are of normal size...The lumina of the renal arteries gape upon section...The adrenals are somewhat smaller than the norm, especially the left one.

ANATOMICAL DIAGNOSIS

Generalized arteriosclerosis with pronounced degree of affection of the cerebral arteries.

Arteriosclerosis of the descending aorta.

Hypertrophy of the right ventricle of the heart.

Multiple foci of yellow cerebromalacia (based on vascular sclerosis) of the left cerebral hemisphere in a stage of resolution and of cystic change.

Fresh hemorrhage into the vascular plexus overlying the corpora quadrigemina.

IMMEDIATE CAUSE OF DEATH

1. The aggravation of the circulatory disturbance of the brain, and

2. Hemorrhage into the arachnoid pia mater in the area of the corpora quadrigemina.

Although the clinical diagnosis of the neurological problems that dominated the final 2 years of Lenin's short but undeniably event-filled life is hardly a mystery, their etiology is. At an age that today would define someone as *in his prime*, Lenin experienced a series of incapacitating strokes, ultimately ending in his death and cutting short his turbulent existence. In 2012, Dr. Harry Vinters, a world-renowned neuropathologist, reviewed the possible causes of Lenin's strange variety of cerebral arteriosclerosis during a historical clinicopathological conference hosted by the VA Maryland Health Care System and the University of Maryland School of Medicine (60). The following discussion draws heavily upon his presentation.

Lenin developed rapidly evolving neurological deficits that left him paralyzed with impaired speech and effectively incapacitated during his final months. Although infections of the central nervous system, such as viral encephalitis, brain abscess, and meningitis, can produce rapidly evolving neurological deficits, there is no evidence that Lenin exhibited signs (e.g., fever) or symptoms (e.g., delirium) typical of such infections.

What about syphilis? Could syphilis have been responsible for his series of strokes? His physicians were concerned enough about that possibility to have treated Lenin with the primitive medication available at the time in spite of several reportedly negative blood tests for syphilis. *Treponema pallidum,* the bacterium responsible for syphilis, does invade the brain, but when it does, it typically attacks small meningeal arteries, not large cerebral vessels of the kind found calcified in Lenin's brain at post-mortem examination. Such meningovascular syphilis can produce regions of chronic cerebral ischemia (61), though usually fairly small ones, which would not present in the catastrophic way that Lenin's neurological deficits evolved. Syphilis also attacks the aorta, causing it to become inflamed and sometimes to balloon outward into an aneurysm (62). Lenin's post-mortem examination apparently did not show evidence of such abnormalities, nor was there evidence of tuberculosis, another infection common in Russia during Lenin's time, which can cause inflammation and thickening of the arteries at the base of the brain (63).

Lenin's neurological disorder was by no means unique among 20th-century world leaders. Woodrow Wilson and Franklin D. Roosevelt both had massive strokes while in office; Roosevelt's was fatal. Winston Churchill and Dwight D. Eisenhower also fell victim to strokes before the end of their terms, though their deficits were minor by comparison (64). None of these other world leaders had a clinical course quite like Lenin's.

Strokes, defined clinically as rapidly progressive, irreversible, nonconvulsive neurological deficits, are grouped into several major subtypes according to their presentation and etiology (Table 11.1). Our understanding of their pathogenesis and the nature of cerebrovascular disease in general has advanced greatly since the

TABLE 11.1

Types of Stroke by Etiology

A. ACUTE STROKE

    1. Central nervous system (brain, spinal cord, retinal) infarction

    2. Intracerebral (parenchymal) hemorrhage

    3. Subarachnoid hemorrhage

    4. Cerebral venous thrombosis

B. SILENT STROKE

    1. Silent brain infarct (may be as frequent as 8–28%)

    2. Silent cerebral hemorrhage (including microhemorrhage)

From reference 60.

1920s (65), thanks to the advent of modern radiographic techniques that enable clinicians to visualize the brain and its vascular supply in astonishing detail (66). None of these techniques was available in Lenin's day. Short of an autopsy, his physicians could only infer the location and the nature of a stroke from a meticulous neurological examination.

The most likely etiology of Comrade Lenin's strokes was a sudden interruption of blood flow to areas of the brain (cerebral ischemia) that evolved through one of several pathways. His autopsy revealed rock-hard cerebral arteries that were nearly bereft of channels through which blood might flow to nourish his brain. There was also systemic arteriosclerosis, though less pronounced elsewhere than in the arteries carrying blood to the brain. Inadequate blood flow to regions of Lenin's brain might have occurred because debris (either cholesterol or clot) dislodged from one artery had traveled to and occluded another cerebral artery. Lenin's autopsy report indicates that at least some of the atheromatous plaques that had formed within his arteries ulcerated, possibly because of hemorrhaging into their lipid cores (Fig. 11.2). When this happens, clot tends to form in the ulcer crater and causes a stroke by occluding the vessel at that site or dislodges (embolizes) and occludes a cerebral artery elsewhere.

An intriguing and poorly understood feature of systemic atherosclerosis is its variable progression within different arterial beds (67). Although Lenin had prominent aortic and coronary atherosclerosis identified at post-mortem examination—a finding highly unusual for a man only in his early 50s—the extent of the lesions identified in these vessels paled in comparison with that found in his cerebral arteries. It was his sclerosed cerebral arteries that were responsible for both his strokes and the cystic cavities that formed in their aftermath, the largest of which developed in the left cerebral hemisphere. Although cerebral infarctions

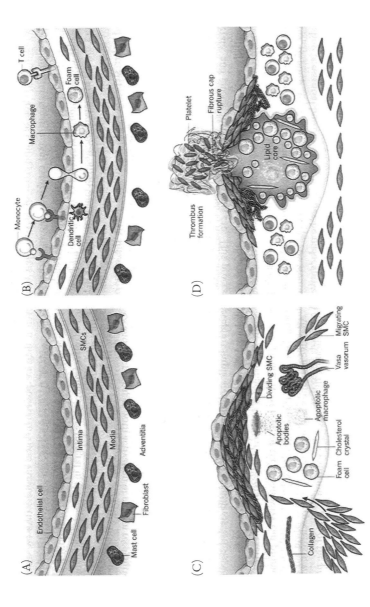

FIGURE 11.2 Stages in the development of atherosclerotic plaques. (A) The three layers of a normal arterial wall: the inner layer, or intima, lined by endothelial cells in direct contact with blood flowing through the lumen of the vessel; the middle layer, or media, containing smooth muscle cells (SMC) embedded in a complex extracellular matrix; and the adventitia, the outer layer, containing mast cells, nerve endings, and nutrient microvessels. (B) The initial phase of atherosclerosis involving adhesion to and then invasion of the intima by inflammatory cells and then uptake of lipid by the inflammatory cells, converting them to "foam cells." (C) Plaque formation involving proliferation of SMCs, accumulation of foam cells, deposition of cholesterol crystals, and invasion by microvessels. (D) Ulceration of a lipid-laden plaque, leading to the formation of a clot in the ulcerated area and occlusion of the vessel lumen. (Reprinted by permission from Macmillan Publishers Ltd., Nature Publishing Group. Libby P, Ridker PM, Hansson GK. Progress and challenges in translating the biology of atherosclerosis. *Nature* 2011;473:317–325)

are sometimes caused by clots released from the inner surface of the heart (cardio-genic emboli), Lenin's autopsy report contains no evidence of such emboli.

Could Lenin's strokes have been cerebral hemorrhages that eventually reab-sorbed, leaving only cystic cavities in their wake? This, too, is unlikely given that Lenin's strokes were unaccompanied by either the sudden, severe headaches typi-cal of cerebral hemorrhages or evidence of an enlarging mass of blood within the brain (68). Cerebral infarctions generally occur because a cerebral artery becomes obstructed by an atherosclerotic plaque or blood clot. Cerebral hemorrhages occur because of the rupture of a defective vessel within the brain—one more often than not part of a vascular malformation, a tumor, or some other intrinsic small vessel abnormality. Some occur because of a systemic clotting disorder, such as a leukemia or low platelet count (thrombocytopenia). Vascular disorders, such as cerebral arteriolosclerosis (sclerosis of small cerebral arteries), are other rare causes of intracerebral bleeds (69, 70), usually though not inevitably accompanied by post-mortem evidence of longstanding hypertension, such as thickening of the wall of the left ventricle of the heart and shrunken kidneys (71, 72), none of which was mentioned in Lenin's autopsy report.

It remains a puzzle as to why a man as young as Lenin and seemingly as vigorous, with few classical risk factors for cerebrovascular disease (73), would develop such severe—indeed rapidly fatal—atherosclerosis. He had migraines, which rarely are associated with paralysis. Although they can cause long-term neurological deficits, migraines rarely if ever cause permanent hemiplegia (74). Furthermore, migraines, even the unusual hemiplegic variant, are not a cause of severe atherosclerosis of the cerebral arteries. With regard to other classic risk factors for cerebrovascu-lar disease, Lenin was a nonsmoker and, judging from his necropsy findings, not hypertensive.

Dimitri Volkogonov, the first researcher to gain access to Lenin's secret Soviet files as director of the Institute of Military History (75), believed that Lenin was "simply destroyed by the strains of power" (76). Prior to the October Revolution, Lenin was accustomed to literary activities, vacationing in the mountains, and Party squabbles in exile, none of which prepared him for the stress of commanding a new government. Could the stress of command have had a role in Lenin's prema-ture atherosclerosis? Certainly, his career as revolutionary leader involved stress, the magnitude of which few of us can even imagine—witness several failed assas-sination attempts. However, stress is difficult to quantify and affects people in different ways. Therefore, invoking it as a risk factor for stroke or, for that matter, any other disorder must be done with caution. Nevertheless, an expanding body of evidence does suggest that psychological stress predisposes to cardiovascular dis-ease, especially atherosclerotic coronary artery disease, as well as cerebrovascular disease (77–84). The precise mechanisms by which stress might contribute to the development of atherosclerosis are poorly understood but are thought to involve invasion of arterial walls by inflammatory cells, particularly monocytes, in response to the influence of an overstimulated hypothalamic-pituitary-adrenal feedback system (85). Indeed, a recent epidemiological study from Japan, examining the role of occupational stress in over 6,000 subjects, found that men with high-strain jobs were nearly three times as likely to suffer a stroke as those with low-strain jobs; this effect was not identified among the women studied (78).

Lenin's father expired at precisely the age our patient did, apparently with similar neurological complaints. Lenin's brother died young of a myocardial infarction and another brother of "stenocardia" (angina) at age 69. A sister had a fatal stroke at the age of 71. Although certainly not conclusive, these findings suggest that there was a family predisposition to atherosclerosis inherited from the father— possibly a familial lipid disorder.

However, Lenin's atherosclerosis was different from what one generally sees in patients with an inherited lipid disorder. His involved the arteries of the brain to a greater extent than those of the heart and exhibited a degree of calcification unprecedented in the experience of Dr. Vinters—a neuropathologist with over three decades devoted to the study of cerebrovascular disorders. In that Lenin's vascular abnormality was so unusual, its etiology most likely was also unusual.

In February 2011, St. Hilaire, Ziegler, Markello, and colleagues published a report in the *New England Journal of Medicine* (86) describing nine persons in three families with markedly calcified arteries of the lower extremities as well as calcification of the joints of the hands and feet. Most of the patients had a history of longstanding pain in the calves and buttocks with exertion (claudication) and painful feet at rest (ischemia). When their personal physicians could not give them a diagnosis, they found their way to Dr. St. Hilaire's Undiagnosed Diseases Program (UDP) at the National Institutes of Health, in search of an explanation for their strange vascular disorder. The UDP team conducted their own comprehensive clinical and radiographic evaluation and then performed genetic studies on the three families. In each family they found a mutation of a gene involved in the calcium metabolic pathway, the NT5E gene, which they believe had a role in causing their patients' arteries and joints to become calcified.

Given the similarity of the disorder described above with that of Lenin (and likely Lenin's family), a final possible explanation for Lenin's highly unusual form of atherosclerosis is an as-yet-undiscovered genetic variant of the disorder described by St. Hilaire and colleagues. Lenin's variant, if it existed, would have been one associated with extensive calcification of the major vessels of the brain, rather than of the legs, and also characterized by longstanding head pain (migraines) rather than leg pain (claudication). This hypothesis could be tested if genetic studies were performed on Lenin's tissues preserved in his mausoleum just outside the Kremlin wall (Fig. 11.3) or on those stored in the Moscow Brain Institute. However, it is not likely that permission to do so will be granted any time soon. If Lenin were alive today and suffering with such a disorder, little could be done to halt, much less reverse, the process by which his cerebral vessels were turned to stone.

While Lenin's health was spiraling downward, Stalin was consolidating his position as Secretary General of the All-Russia Communist Party. At the end of September 1922, the two came into open conflict over principles concerning the organization of the future Soviet Union. "Stalin," Lenin railed, "is in rather too much of a hurry... [He] has unlimited authority in his hands, and I am not sure whether he will always be capable of using that authority with sufficient caution." In January 1923, Lenin went further, charging that "Stalin is too rude, and this defect, although quite tolerable in our midst and in dealing among us Communists, becomes intolerable in a Secretary General. That is why I suggest that the comrades think about a way of removing Stalin from the post and appointing another man in his stead who in all other respects differs from Comrade Stalin in having

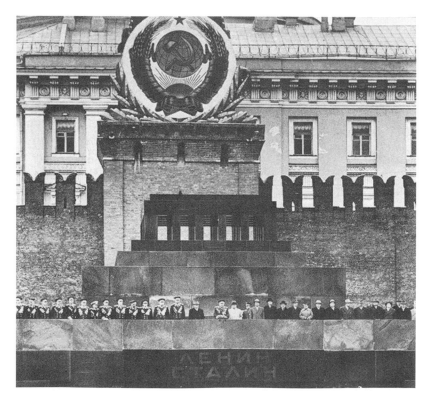

FIGURE 11.3 Lenin's mausoleum outside the Kremlin wall in Moscow.

only one advantage, namely, that of being more tolerant, more loyal, more polite and more considerate to the comrades, less capricious, etc." By March the struggle had become mortal, with Stalin having the upper hand as the Secretary General in control of both the Party apparatus and Lenin's medical care. By then Lenin's health was in precipitous decline. However, he had rallied before, and if he were able to return to politics once more, even briefly, Stalin's political liquidation would have been certain (87). Therefore, when Lenin begged for potassium cyanide to end his misery following his third major stroke (9, 88), there are those who believe that Stalin saw to it that his plea did not go unanswered. Given Lenin's terminal seizures, which are characteristic of acute cyanide poisoning and atypical of strokes, not to mention the subsequent mysterious deaths of numerous members of Stalin's inner circle (e.g., Mikhail Frunze, Valerian Kuybyshev, and Maxim Gorky), cyanide poisoning must be added to the list of potential proximate causes of Lenin's death.

Many have wondered whether the Soviets would have followed a different path if Lenin had not died in 1924—one less militaristic and politically sterile than that which evolved under Stalin. There has been speculation that if Lenin had not succumbed to premature cerebrovascular disease, his New Economic Policy allowing peasants to work in part for themselves, and permitting a degree of latitude in cultural life, would have continued and led to a more tolerant order of things (89). Others are convinced that no good could possibly have come from a man "concerned more with destruction—terrible, total, universal and merciless destruction—than creation of a new world" (90). We can never know which path history might have followed had Lenin's vessels not turned to stone, for at the height of his power, his life, having flamed for its allotted time, withered and died forever (91).

References

1. Payne R. *The Life and Death of Lenin*. New York: Simon and Schuster, 1964:24.
2. Ibid., dust cover.
3. Ibid., p. 28.
4. Volkogonov D. *Lenin. A New Biography* (translated by H. Shukman). New York: The Free Press, 1996:326.
5. Service R. *Lenin. A Biography*. Cambridge, MA: Belknap Press of Harvard University Press, 2000:172.
6. Ibid., p. 177.
7. Ibid., p. 81.
8. Op. cit. Volkogonov, p. 343.
9. Ibid., p. 420.
10. Op. cit. Service, p. 391.
11. Ibid., p. 434.

12. Op. cit. Volkogonov, p. 432.
13. Op. cit. Service, p. 492.
14. Op. cit. Volkogonov, p. 3.
15. Op. cit. Service, pp. 31–32.
16. Ibid., p. 190.
17. Ibid., pp. 101–102, 108.
18. Ibid., p. 89.
19. Ibid., pp. 112, 456.
20. Ibid., p. 150.
21. Ibid., pp. 163, 188.
22. Ibid., p. 186.
23. Ibid., pp. 368–369.
24. Op. cit. Volkogonov, pp. 226–229.
25. Op. cit. Service, p. 445.
26. Op. cit. Volkogonov, p. 8.
27. Ibid., p. 5.
28. Ibid., p. 2.
29. Op. cit. Service, pp. 48–49.
30. Ibid., p. 230.
31. Ibid., p. 86.
32. Op. cit. Volkogonov, p. 29.
33. Op. cit. Service, p. 100.
34. Ibid., pp. 197–198.
35. Ibid., p. 415.
36. Ibid., p. 148.
37. Ibid., p. 117.
38. Ibid., p. 187.
39. Ibid., pp. 33, 64, 108, 164, 188, 211, 373.
40. Op. cit. Volkogonov, p. 35.
41. Op. cit. Service, p. 263.
42. Ibid., p. 365.
43. Ibid., p. 99.
44. Ibid., p. 447.
45. Op. cit. Volkogonov, pp. 410–411.
46. Ibid., pp. 138–139.
47. Ibid., p. xxxvii.
48. Op. cit. Service, p. 61.
49. Ibid., p. 72.
50. Ibid., p. 83.
51. Ibid., p. 435.
52. Op. cit. Volkogonov, p. 273.
53. Ibid., p. 427.
54. Op. cit. Service, p. 158.
55. Ibid., p. 443.
56. Ibid., p. 444.
57. Op. cit. Volkogonov, p. 142.
58. Op. cit. Payne, p. 595.

59. Ibid., pp. 637–640.

60. Vinters H, Lurie, L, Mackowiak PA. Vessels of stone. Lenin's "circulatory disturbance of the brain." *Human Pathol* 2013; Feb 18. pii:S0046–8177(12)00445–5.

61. Vinters HV. Infectious and inflammatory diseases causing dementia. In Esiri MM, Lee VM-Y, Trojanowski JQ, eds. *The Neuropathology of Dementia*, 2nd ed. Cambridge: Cambridge University Press, 2004:472–496.

62. Virmani R, Burke AP. Nonatherosclerotic diseases of the aorta and miscellaneous diseases of the main pulmonary arteries and large veins. In Silver MD, Gotlieb AI, Schoen FJ, eds. *Cardiovascular Pathology*, 3rd ed. New York/Edinburgh: Churchill Livingstone, 2001:107–137.

63. Lammie GA, Hewlett RH, Schoeman JF, Donald PR. Tuberculous cerebrovascular disease: A review. *J Infection* 2009;59:156–166.

64. Friedlander WJ. About three old men: an inquiry into how cerebral arteriosclerosis has altered world politics. A neurologist's view. *Stroke* 1972;3:467–473.

65. Vinters HV. Cerebrovascular disease—Practical issues in surgical and autopsy pathology. *Current Topics in Pathology* 2001;95:51–99.

66. Chalela JA, Kidwell CS, Nentwich LM, et al. Magnetic resonance imaging and computed tomography in emergency assessment of patients with suspected acute stroke: a prospective comparison. *Lancet* 2007;369:293–298.

67. Adraktas DD, Brasic N, Furtado AD, et al. Carotid atherosclerosis does not predict coronary, vertebral, or aortic atherosclerosis in patients with acute stroke symptoms. *Stroke* 2010;41:1604–1609.

68. Qureshi AI, Mendelow AD, Hanley DF. Intracerebral haemorrhage. *Lancet* 2009;373:1632–1644.

69. Vinters HV. Cerebral amyloid angiopathy—a critical review. *Stroke* 1987;18:311–324.

70. Verbeek MM, de Waal RMW, Vinters HV, eds. *Cerebral Amyloid Angiopathy in Alzheimer's Disease and Related Disorders*. Dordrecht/Boston: Kluwer Academic, 2000.

71. Lammie GA, Brannan F, Slattery J, Warlow C. Nonhypertensive cerebral small-vessel disease. An autopsy study. *Stroke* 1997;28:2222–2229.

72. Lammie GA. Hypertensive cerebral small vessel disease and stroke. *Brain Pathol* 2002;12:358–370.

73. Yasaka M, Yamaguchi T, Shichiri M. Distribution of atherosclerosis and risk factors in atherothrombotic occlusion. *Stroke* 1993;24:206–211.

74. Russell MB, Ducros A. Sporadic and familial hemiplegic migraine: pathophysiological mechanisms, clinical characteristics, diagnosis, and management. *Lancet Neurol* 2011;10:457–470.

75. Op. cit. Volkogonov, p. xxv.

76. Ibid., p. 436.

77. Steptoe A, Kivimaki M. Stress and cardiovascular disease. *Nat Rev Cardiol* 2012. doi:10.1038/nrcardio.2012.45.

78. Tsutsumi A, Kayaba K, Ishikawa S. Impact of occupational stress on stroke across occupational classes and genders. *Social Science and Medicine* 2011;72:1652–1658.

79. Suadincani P, Andersen LL, Holtermann A, et al. Perceived psychological pressure at work, social class, and risk of stroke: a 30-year follow-up in Copenhagen male study. *J Occupational Environ Med* 2011;53:1388–1395.

80. Guiraud V, Amor MB, Mas JL, Touze E. Triggers of ischemic stroke: a systematic review. *Stroke* 2010;41:2669–2677.

81. Kornerup H, Osler M, Boysen G, et al. Major life events increase the risk of stroke but not of myocardial infarction: results from the Copenhagen City heart study. *Eur J Cardiovasc Prevention Rehab* 2010;17:113–118.

82. Jood K, Redfors P, Rosengren A, et al. Self-perceived psychological stress and ischemic stroke: a case-control study. *BMC Med* 2009;7:53.

83. Surtees PG, Wainwright NW, Luben RN, et al. Psychological distress, major depressive disorder, and risk of stroke. *Neurol* 2008;70:788–794.

84. Harmsen P, Lappas G, Rosengren A, Wilhelmsen L. Long-term risk factors for stroke: twenty-eight years of follow-up of 7457 middle-aged men in Goteborg, Sweden. *Stroke* 2006;37:1663–1667.

85. Gu H-F, Tang C-K, Yang Y-Z. Psychological stress, immune response, and atherosclerosis. *Atherosclerosis* 2012, doi:10:1016/j.atherosclerosis.2012.01.021.

86. St. Hilaire CS, Ziegler SG, Markello TC, et al. NT5E mutations and arterial calcifications. *N Engl J Med* 2011;364:432–442.

87. Lewin M. *Lenin's Last Struggle*. London: Faber and Faber, 1969:79–83, 145–151.

88. Op. cit. Volkogonov, p. 426.

89. Ibid., p. xxvii.

90. Op. cit. Payne, p. 29.

91. *The Iliad*, Book XXI, l. 15–18.

What remains to this day as the essence of his persona is, to my mind, one of the truly great natural tenor voices of the past century...a voice which, incidentally, not only made an impact on me, but also on many of my tenor colleagues, like Luciano Pavarotti and José Carreras.

PLÁCIDO DOMINGO (1)

12 Fatal Zest for Living

ACCORDING TO NO less an authority than Arturo Toscanini, this patient had "the greatest natural tenor voice of the 20th Century" (2). He sang "with purity and power, with conviction and lucidity...Not a note was neglected or over-emphasized." He might have been a "new Caruso" had he not been seduced by the glitter and fanfare of Hollywood. "I'm young. I have time," he reasoned in postponing his dream of an operatic career while pursuing one in film. Unfortunately, he had far less time than he imagined. In fewer than 10 years Hollywood would make him famous, but also leave him hopelessly confused and insecure. By his 30s his health was gone, victimized by an abundance of flesh, crash diets, and alcohol. He was dead before reaching his 39th birthday (3).

The patient was born on January 31, 1921, in South Philadelphia, in a bedroom above the grocery store his maternal grandfather had given to his parents. He was an only child, with a warm and bubbly personality, whose two great loves were music and sports. When he was 12, his parents took him to his first opera, *Aida*. Afterward, nothing excited him as much as opera (4).

The patient's mother had hoped he might become a doctor or a lawyer. However, when she and her husband first heard him sing, they were moved to tears by the raw beauty of his voice and realized that singing, not medicine or law, was their son's true calling. But, he was only 16 then and had to wait another 2 years for his voice to mature before beginning his formal training. In the meantime, he worked hard with weights and pulleys and a stationary bicycle to tone his muscular body and to resist a tendency to gain weight (4).

In the summer of 1940, when he was 19, the patient decided it was time to begin his voice lessons. His first instructor, Irene Williams, was a soprano who had sung with Nelson Eddy during his pre-Hollywood days. For $5 per lesson, she coached the patient in repertoire (5). Instruction in voice production and technique would come later. Under her tutelage, he made such remarkable progress that on auditioning with Serge Koussevitzky 2 years later, the legendary conductor of the Boston Symphony exclaimed: "Yours is a voice such as is heard only once in a hundred years" (6).

Koussevitzky took the patient to Tanglewood and placed him under the direction of strict taskmasters of the likes of conductors Leonard Bernstein, Lukas Foss, and Boris Goldovsky (7). The patient labored under them for 8 to 10 hours a day and in 6 weeks was ready for his operatic debut, as Fenton, in Otto Nicolai's *The Merry Wives of Windsor*. The critics rated his performance as that of a singer "whose superb natural voice has few equals among tenors of the day in quality, warmth and power (8)...a real find of the season... [a singer who] would have no difficulty one day being asked to join the Metropolitan Opera" (9).

The patient's operatic career, however, would have to wait; the Army had other plans for him. In spite of partial blindness in his left eye that had developed in the aftermath of a convulsion suffered as a baby, he received a letter from his local draft board in December 1942 instructing him to report to Miami for basic training (10).

Army life was torture for the patient. "He was a great big boy who enjoyed life to the hilt...and the Army was dull!" It robbed him of his vitality and his zest for living. His solution, which was to become his standard procedure for dealing with moments of crisis and depression, was to overeat—two and a half chickens in one sitting, for example. Though only 5'7½" tall (18), he ballooned to 260 lbs (118 kg) and became an embarrassment to his unit (11).

In January 1945, after nearly 3 years in the Army, mostly spent singing in plays performed at various military bases, the patient was granted a medical discharge for "an ear infection and post-nasal drip." Three months later, he married the sister of an Army buddy. The patient was 24, his bride 22. They would have four children, two boys and two girls, and later die within 3 months of each other (12).

After leaving the Army, the patient worked hard on vocal technique under a host of distinguished teachers and by 1947 appeared "unmistakably destined for a major operatic career." However, a stunning performance as a substitute for the famous Italian tenor Ferruccio Tagliavini at the Hollywood Bowl in Los Angeles would prove to be a turning point in his career, one that would prevent him from ever appearing at La Scala, the Metropolitan, or any other renowned operatic stage. Upon hearing the performance, MGM mogul Louis B. Mayer recognized immediately that the talented, handsome, and vivacious young tenor had all of the qualities of a cinematic star. Three days later, he signed the patient to a contract with MGM that included a $10,000 bonus, an initial salary of $750 per week for a period of 20 weeks the first year, $1,250 per week the second year, $1,400 per week the third, and so on, to $2,750 per week in the seventh year. With what was then a small fortune, the patient began "eating the best food in the best restaurants, drinking the most expensive wines and champagnes, and wearing the best clothes" (13).

When he arrived on the set for his first film, *That Midnight Kiss*, weighing 200 lbs (90.7 kg), the patient was told that because the camera lens added extra pounds to an actor, he would have to lose approximately 30 lbs (13.6 kg) before shooting could begin. He resisted at first, explaining that a singer "needed poundage [below the diaphragm] to be in best voice." Eventually, he acquiesced and began what would be the first of countless, exhausting battles to lose weight for the camera. After 4 months of dieting and exercise under the direction of a physical trainer, he lost 31 lbs and was ready to begin work on his first film (11).

The movie-going public, accustomed to the archetypal portly tenor, had never witnessed the combination of a sublime tenor voice emerging from a handsome face and winning personality such as this patient presented. He was so handsome, in fact, that for the first time in motion picture history, the camera remained on close-up of a classical singer for the full length of an aria. However, the patient's looks proved to be a curse as well as a blessing. Had he been "cross-eyed or hare-lipped or possessed some other factor that would have disqualified him from making movies," he might well have been one of the star opera singers of his time (14).

With the release of *That Midnight Kiss*, the patient became an immediate star (15). A series of films followed in quick succession, which in just 2 years made him the most popular singer in America.

Unfortunately, as the patient's fame soared, so did his insecurity (13). Alcohol became his refuge. Whereas formerly he had limited himself to a glass of red wine with meals, as the pressures of stardom increased, so did his consumption of alcohol. In addition to ever-increasing quantities of wine, he began drinking Scotch, which actor David Niven had introduced to him while filming *The Toast of New Orleans* in 1949–50. While working on the film, he made a brave effort to control his drinking and to manage his weight by not eating lunch and exercising instead. However, in the long run, skipping meals and working out would not be enough, and he became increasingly reliant on crash diets, pills, and injections to control his weight (16).

In 1952 a series of unfortunate investments by the patient's manager left the tenor not just financially destitute but in debt to the government for more than

$250,000 in back taxes. The collapse of his finances, a break with his manager, and then an intense disagreement with management during work on a new film, *The Student Prince*, brought the volatile performer to the verge of collapse. He walked off the set, was fired by MGM, and then sued for breach of contract. He went into seclusion and once again sought refuge in food and alcohol (17).

After 2 years of self-imposed exile, the patient agreed to appear in the premiere of a new CBS television spectacular, *Shower of Stars*, scheduled for September 1954. Massively overweight and self-conscious over his appearance, he decided to return to his crash diet routine, hoping to get into shape, at least marginally, for his television debut. He entered Las Encinas Hospital in Pasadena under the care of the head of the sanatorium, Dr. F. M. Briggs, where he subsisted on a diet of one grapefruit for breakfast, a boiled egg and black coffee for lunch, and a light snack for dinner. He also managed to stop drinking, and by the time he reported to the CBS studios, edgy and exhausted, he had succeeded in reducing his weight from 265 lbs (120 kg) to 225 lbs (102 kg) (18).

When the patient began work on *Serenade*, his final American film, with Warner Bros., in late 1955, he had again ballooned to nearly 260 lbs (118 kg). He managed to lose 60 lbs (23 kg) by the time the film was completed. However, by then, it was apparent that the matinee idol looks of his MGM days were fading (19).

A scathing review of *Serenade* by *Time* magazine, coupled with modest ticket sales, plunged the patient into another bout of depression. He again began to drink heavily. Then, in May 1957, he decided to try his luck in Europe and sailed with his family for Naples, never to return to America (20).

A new (Italian) film, *Seven Hills of Rome*, promised relief from his financial difficulties. For starring in the film, the patient was to receive a fee of $200,000 plus 30 percent of the gross. However, at 243 lbs (110.2 kg), he first had to undergo yet another crash diet to prepare for the camera. This time he was to be admitted to the Salvador Mundi Hospital under the care of Dr. Albert T. W. Simeons, reputedly one of Europe's leading weight-reduction experts. The secret to Simeons' special method for reducing weight was to inject patients with the urine of a pregnant woman "to raise the rate of metabolism to burn excess calories." In response to these injections, along with a 500-calorie daily diet supplemented with vitamin injections, the patient shed 30 lbs (13.6 kg) in just 9 days and another 44 lbs (20 kg) over the course of 3 months. By the time filming was finished, he weighed a mere 169 lbs (76.6 kg) and looked "tired and drawn." With no specific goal to pursue once work on the film had been completed, he drifted into depression and resumed his heavy drinking (21).

In January 1958, while descending steps into the garden at Lana Turner's home outside of London, the patient slipped, fell, and badly bruised his ribs. Three days later, while touring in Germany, he developed pain and swelling in his right leg. When examined by a Dr. Frederic Fruhwein, he was informed that he had high blood pressure as well as phlebitis (an inflamed blood clot) in his right leg. Fruhwein warned him of the danger of a pulmonary embolism and predicted that if he continued his current lifestyle, he would be dead in a year (3).

Utterly exhausted following a scheduled concert in Stuttgart, the patient cancelled remaining appearances and returned to Rome to be admitted into the Valle Giulia, a private clinic owned and supervised by a Dr. Guido Moricca. He was immediately placed on total bed rest and given "a course of injections to relieve the swelling and pain" in his phlebitic leg (3).

The patient resumed his interrupted concert tour against Moricca's advice, after resting for a month, first in the Valle Giulia clinic and then at home. With the aid of a cane and his leg wrapped tightly in a rubber stocking, he limped his way to the airport, flew to London, and then proceeded by train to Bristol, where the tour was scheduled to resume (22).

Toward the end of his Bristol recital, the patient was in so much pain that he finished the performance leaning on his cane. After singing three habitual encores, he hobbled to his dressing room, where he was given a pain-killing injection. He pressed on to Newcastle, Brighton, and Bradford, singing one concert after another, each time receiving a pain-killing injection before performing (22).

In April 1958, the patient developed a sore throat and other symptoms of a cold. He was in Hamburg at the time and had been drinking a great deal of beer while singing various arias from *Otello* over and over again until the early hours of the morning. When examined by an ear, nose, and throat specialist and then by a second physician, he was informed that he had an enlarged heart and a badly damaged liver. They advised him to stop drinking immediately. The patient cancelled his Hamburg concert and returned to Rome, where an examination by his personal physician, Professor Guiseppe Stradone, confirmed the German doctors' diagnoses. The ailing tenor had an enlarged heart and a bad liver. He was also suffering from bronchitis and persistent inflammation of his right leg. What's more, "his blood pressure was 290 [sic]" (23).

Given his financial difficulties, the patient agreed to appear in another film, *For the First Time*. Weighing 260 lbs (118 kg), however, he was in no condition to face the camera and decided to embark on yet another crash diet. On May 28, 1958, he entered Walchensee, a posh sanatorium for alcoholics and overweight people situated in the Bavarian Alps, under the care of Dr. Fruhwein, the same German physician who 4 months earlier had diagnosed his phlebitis and hypertension. Fruhwein's plan was for the patient to undergo 2 weeks of Megaphen-induced "twilight sleep therapy," during which he was to be fed intravenously. The treatment was designed not just to reduce a patient's weight but also to provide a period of rest that would allow him to awaken refreshed physically as well as mentally. Shortly after attempting to induce twilight sleep, Fruhwein realized that the standard dose of Megaphen was having no effect on his patient and feared that given the tenor's sick liver and enlarged heart, high blood pressure, and phlebitis, sleep therapy induced by a stronger dose of the drug might prove fatal. He therefore cancelled the twilight sleep therapy and instead placed the patient on a program consisting of a strict diet and vigorous exercise under close supervision. In just 8 weeks, the patient lost 45 lbs (20.4 kg) and returned to Rome feeling healthy (24).

Although in excellent voice in *For the First Time*, the patient looked tired and edgy and older than his 37 years. Gone was the vitality that had taken Hollywood by storm. While working on the film, he managed to control his drinking, but the moment the cameras stopped rolling, he returned to the bottle (25).

The New Year found the patient in poor health. An electrocardiogram taken by cardiologist Loredano Dalla Torre reportedly showed "damage to the myocardium and coronary insufficiency." Two months later the patient complained of chest pain and was admitted to the Valle Giulia clinic, where "a minor heart attack" was diagnosed. His phlebitis was also troubling him; he was overweight and had a blood pressure of "290". Dr. Stradone gave him medication for his phlebitis and ordered complete rest for 2 weeks. Immediately after being discharged from the clinic, the patient began rehearsing for a series of new recordings (26).

Then, late one rainy evening following an argument with his wife, the patient stormed out of the house inebriated. After spending most of the night out of doors, he woke the next morning with a fever. He was taken to the Valle Giulia clinic, where double pneumonia complicated by a pulmonary embolus was diagnosed. Following "a course of heavy doses of antibiotics," he was discharged in late August to resume work on an interrupted recording of *Desert Song* (27).

When offered an opportunity to star in a new film, *Laugh Clown Laugh*, the patient decided to re-enter the Valle Giulia clinic and once again undergo Dr. Moricca's weight-reducing program. He was admitted on September 25, 1959, weighing 253.5 lbs (115 kg). Dr. Fruhwein had forwarded his medical file from Walchensee with a clear warning for Dr. Moricca that under no circumstances should he subject the singer to sleep therapy, given the condition of his liver and the danger of a blood clot embolizing from his leg to his lungs with prolonged immobilization. Moricca ignored his German colleague and proceeded with sleep therapy as planned (28).

On Tuesday evening, October 6, his twilight sleep therapy completed, the patient performed one of his favorite arias, *"E lucevan le steile,"* for the hospital staff. The following morning he spoke briefly by phone with his wife and his agent, Sam Steinman. Shortly before noon Mario Lanza (né Alfred "Freddie" Cacozza)

(Fig. 12.1) was found reclining on the divan in his room, motionless, extremely pale, with his head turned to the side (28). Silent forever was "a voice such as is heard only once in a hundred years" (6).

Lanza's medical problems, of which there were many, were largely products of a zest for living taken to the extreme. He "overate, over-drank, overslept, over-did things generally" (29). The overeating, perhaps his most self-destructive activity, one that had haunted him since his childhood, was for him an enjoyment and an escape, an expression of his *joie de vivre,* and an outlet for his bubbly personality (4).

When admitted to the Valle Giulia clinic in Rome just before he died, Lanza weighed 253.5 lbs (28). At a height of only 5'7½", few would argue that at that weight he was obese, or that his obesity was, at least in part, responsible for many of his health problems. Like obese people in general, he would have been prone to cardiovascular disease, hypertension, thrombophlebitis, and steatohepatitis (fatty liver). Obesity is also associated with insulin resistance, diabetes mellitus, obstructive sleep apnea, gastroesophageal reflux disorder (GERD), degenerative joint disease (osteoarthritis), surgical complications, polycystic ovaries, and impaired

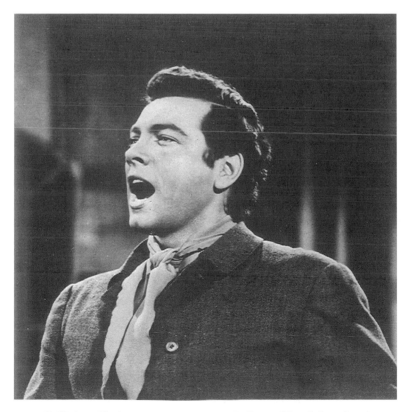

FIGURE 12.1 Publicity still of Lanza in a scene from *The Toast of New Orleans* (1951).

immunity (30–33). What more evidence could one ask for as proof that obesity is bad for one's health or that it had a critical role in Lanza's premature death?

Webster's Collegiate Dictionary defines obesity as "a condition characterized by excessive body fat." Nutritionists and public health experts have a more objective definition—a body mass index (BMI) of 30 or more (calculated as weight in kilograms divided by the height in meters squared) (34). According to the Centers for Disease Control and Prevention, over one third of the adult U.S. population meets the latter definition for obesity. Over 6 percent of the population has a BMI of 40 or more (34), placing them in the "morbidly obese" category—obesity so potentially dangerous to their health that they qualify immediately for drastic weight-reduction measures such as bariatric surgery (see below) (35). At his heaviest, Lanza's BMI was 40.1.

Obesity, however, is not as simple a concept as one might imagine. If excess body fat is primarily truncal as opposed to predominantly abdominal (the classic "beer belly" distribution), being obese is associated with little excess health risk or reduced lifespan (36). Moreover, because muscle has a positive effect on the metabolism of glucose and fat, the increased muscle mass of patients like Lanza (11) tends to mitigate the adverse effects of obesity on health (37). Although on average obese persons have shorter lifespans than lean persons, when other potential risk factors are taken into account (for example, smoking, diabetes, or hypertension), there is little difference between obese and lean subjects with regard to mortality (38, 39).

Treatments for obesity are likely as old as civilized concepts of health and beauty. The ancient Greeks' approach to obesity, which they called *diaita*, involved an intervention directed at the whole way of life rather than a narrow weight-loss regimen focused primarily on diet. Over the centuries, endless numbers of "new" weight-loss schemes have emerged and then faded into obscurity, only to re-emerge under different names. Today, for example, diets guaranteed to remove excess fat include the Cabbage Soup diet, the Grapefruit diet, the Three-Day diet, the One-Day diet, the Scarsdale diet, the Zone diet, the South Beach diet, the F-Plan diet, the GI diet, the Atkins, the Dukan, and the MacDougal plans, and so on (40).

For those who are unhappy or unsuccessful with diets in relieving them of their (real or imagined) abundance of flesh, there are hormones and pills that promise to curb their appetite, enhance their thermogenesis (fat burning), inhibit protein breakdown, boost a feeling of fullness, block the absorption of calories and fat, and suppress compulsive eating by elevating one's mood. And then there is surgery—*bariatric* (from the Greek *baros*, "weight") surgery to excise excess fat and to limit the intake or absorption of calories by shrinking the stomach or bypassing portions of the small intestine (41).

None of these interventions are any more effective in the long term than those directed against Lanza's obesity. Although successful dieters initially lose 5 to 10 percent of their weight on any number of modern diets, the weight almost always comes back. In fact, according to a recent report by the American Psychological Association summarizing the results of an analysis of 31 diet studies, after 2 years of dieting, up to two thirds of dieters weighed more than they did before they began dieting (42). Even bariatric surgery rarely produces sustained weight loss. Moreover, improvements in mortality associated with such surgery have been shown to be unrelated to this kind of weight loss (38, 43). In addition, whereas weight loss by whatever means has been shown to ameliorate diabetes and other risk factors for cardiovascular disease (44–47), paradoxically, in most epidemiological studies, it has also been shown to be associated with an increased incidence of cardiovascular events, even among participants who are obese at baseline (48–51). Likewise, lifestyle interventions combined with anti-obesity medications have either shown no effect (52) or in some cases an increase in cardiovascular events in the drug treatment group (53). Starvation diets appear to be particularly dangerous in this regard by predisposing patients to potentially fatal cardiac arrhythmias (54). Whether Lanza's repetitive drastic dieting was especially deleterious to his health by amplifying the reported diet-associated risks of muscle wastage, fractures, cancer, and cardiovascular disease (55) is not known.

Because Lanza's biographies give only a limited number of his systolic pressures, the full extent of his hypertension is uncertain. Today, when blood pressures are recorded, two numbers are given—the systolic pressure, a peak pressure coinciding with cardiac contraction (i.e., *systole*), and a trough pressure coinciding with cardiac relaxation (i.e., *diastole*). In April 1958, almost a year and a half before he died, and again a year later, he had a systolic pressure of 290 mm Hg (22, 26). His diastolic pressures are not available.

In the 1950s, diastolic hypertension was regarded as "more important" than systolic hypertension (56). Therefore, if Lanza's diastolic pressures were normal or near normal, there would have been a tendency to ignore them and also to minimize the danger of his systolic hypertension. This might explain why his physicians, who would have been aware of the capacity of hypertension to damage cerebral and cardiac blood vessels, prescribed none of the standard treatments for hypertension of the day, except for aggressive weight reduction.

In the 1950s, such treatments varied according to the stage of the hypertension. In the "uncomplicated phase," patients were "told of the lack of significance of blood pressure levels and fluctuations, and that high pressures are not necessarily precursors of vascular accidents." At this stage, neither salt restriction, medications, nor any other measures were recommended. Lanza's physicians may well have regarded his hypertension as "uncomplicated" and therefore chose not to prescribe treatments reserved for "symptomatic" patients, which included sedatives such as phenobarbital (Lanza received this medication periodically but in conjunction with weight-reduction programs) and rauwolfia alkaloids such as reserpine. Chlorothiazide diuretics were not recommended in uncomplicated hypertension because it was thought that they "rarely influence the blood pressure when used alone unless an abnormal degree of water and electrolyte depletion is produced." Moreover, in patients with advanced myocardial damage or angina pectoris, both of which Lanza was thought to have had, antihypertensives were discouraged because they were believed to increase the risk of vascular accidents in such patients (56).

Lanza drank heavily, if sporadically, during his final decade, and a "badly damaged liver" diagnosed in Hamburg in April 1958 (23) was likely caused by his alcohol abuse. Nevertheless, it is also possible that his massive obesity had a role in his liver failure by producing nonalcoholic steatohepatitis (fatty liver), a disorder already known to physicians of the 1950s, if not yet by the acronym "NASH." Interestingly, at that time, the direct toxicity of alcohol for hepatocytes (liver cells) was not yet fully appreciated. According to a leading 1950s textbook, "it is still not certain that the pathological changes [seen in various organs in chronic alcoholics] are due to alcohol, related vitamin lack or dietary deficiency . . . The role of alcohol in the causation of hepatic cirrhosis is not clear, for similar cirrhosis is seen in abstainers" (57).

In January 1958, Lanza fell while descending stairs leading into the garden at Lana Turner's home, badly bruising his ribcage (3). Three days later, pain in the right leg heralded the onset of thrombophlebitis. Whether Lanza's thrombosed vein was the result of a leg injury also sustained in the fall or one more complication of his morbid obesity is unknown.

In the 1950s, as in the present, thrombophlebitis was recognized as a potentially lethal condition requiring aggressive therapy. In the acute phase, both active and passive motion of the affected limb were contraindicated. Thrombectomy (surgical removal of the clot) was encouraged, especially for "noninflammatory thrombosis" of large veins. When distal segments of superficial veins, such as the long or short saphenous or deep veins of the calf, were thrombosed, proximal ligation was often performed. For more proximal clots, ligation of the inferior vena cava was the recommended treatment. Local heat, elastic stockings, and anticoagulants were also used, both to hasten resorption of the thrombus and to prevent its further propagation (58).

In April 1959, Lanza complained of chest pain diagnosed as a "minor heart attack" (26). As noted above, his systolic pressure was then 290 mm Hg. In the 1950s, the standard treatment for myocardial infarctions called for complete physical and mental rest for 3 to 6 weeks and then limited activity for an additional 2 months. Immediate management included morphine sulfate for pain, oxygen for dyspnea, aminophylline for additional analgesia, atropine sulfate and quinidine for arrhythmia prophylaxis, and digitalis for congestive failure and atrial tachyarrhythmias. Nitroglycerine was regarded as "hazardous in the acute phase of acute myocardial infarction" and therefore was not recommended (59). Lanza's treatment consisted of a reducing diet and complete rest for 2 weeks. Although an electrocardiogram taken 2 months earlier (Fig. 12.2) reportedly revealed "damage of the myocardium and coronary insufficiency," the tracing presented in a book by Lanza's son (60) is, in fact, normal, raising the possibility that several "heart attacks" diagnosed during his final months were misdiagnosed.

Of the myriad weight-loss programs to which Lanza was subjected to enhance his physical appearance before the camera, two were potentially life-threatening. In May 1958, while still suffering from thrombophlebitis of the right leg, he was admitted to the Walchensee sanatorium to receive treatment for obesity and alcohol addiction. The treatment regimen was to consist of 2 weeks of "twilight sleep" induced by Megaphen, during which he was to be fed intravenously until permitted to awaken "refreshed both physically and mentally." Fortunately for Lanza, Dr. Fruhwein quickly aborted the treatment and possibly averted a fatal pulmonary embolism when he realized that his patient was suffering from an enlarged heart, abnormally high blood pressure, and thrombophlebitis (24).

In mid-1957, Lanza turned to Dr. Simeons of the Salvatore Mundi International Hospital in Rome for treatment of his obesity (21). Simeons' program, one recently revived by self-made millionaire Kevin Trudeau in his book *The Weight Loss Cure* (61), consisted of daily doses of the female sex hormone human chorionic gonadotropin (hCG) in the form of human pregnancy urine and a 500-calorie-per-day diet consisting of "100 gm of lean meat, a normal helping of leafy vegetables, an unsweetened rusk and an apple or the equivalent in fruit, with salt and fluids *ad lib*" (62). Simeons believed, as do current advocates of his regimen, that hCG "renders abnormal fat deposits in the abdomen, thighs, etc. readily available, enabling the obese to live comfortably on 500 calories a day for several weeks" without suffering intolerable pangs of hunger. Although several of Simeons' contemporaries found hCG no more effective than placebo (63), the hormone recently has been shown to have thyroid-stimulating activity due to its molecular homology with thyroid-stimulating hormone (TSH), and when present in the circulation in sufficient quantity and duration, it is capable of inducing the hyperthyroid state (64). Following its administration, the coagulation cascade is also activated with slight elevations of clotting factors II, V, VII, VIII, and IX and fibrinogen (65), which might have had an ancillary role in Lanza's refractory thrombophlebitis.

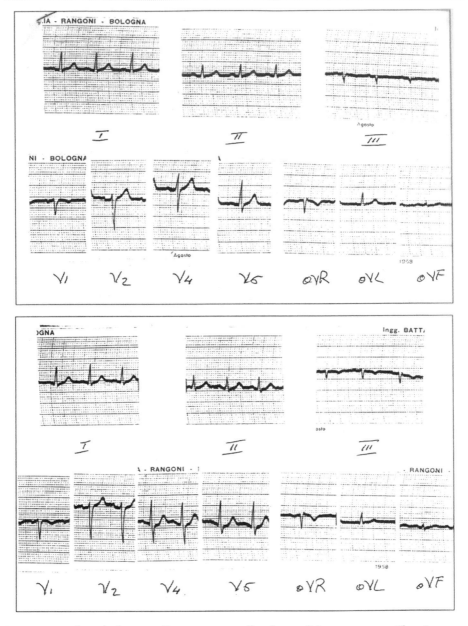

FIGURE 12.2 Lanza's electrocardiogram, supposedly taken on February 14, 1959. Close inspection reveals that it is labeled "Ragoni-Bologna," and although presented in Lanza's son's book as his father's electrocardiogram, is more likely that of some other patient.

Whether Lanza was injected with quantities of hCG sufficient to induce thyrotoxicosis while under Simeons' care is unknown. However, in his first 9 days at the Salvatore Mundi International Hospital, he lost an astonishing 30 lbs and then another 44 lbs in the ensuing 3 months, leaving him "tired and drawn" in appearance (21). Whether he received additional hCG injections during subsequent weight-loss programs is, likewise, unknown.

Lanza died suddenly the morning of October 7, 1959, when just 38 years old. The particular physical catastrophe responsible for silencing forever a voice judged "black and warm and dead on pitch...strong as a pillar from top to bottom (3)...such as is heard only once in a hundred years" (6) will never be known. No autopsy was performed (28), and what remains of Lanza's medical record is far too meager to reveal the secret of his premature death. All we know for certain is that his health was already unraveling when he entered the Valle Giulia clinic on September 25, 1959, to rest and to lose weight. The day before he died he was fit enough to sing "*E lucevan le stelle*" from *Tosca* for the clinic staff and the next morning to converse with his wife and his agent on the telephone, before being found "reclining in the divan [in his room], motionless, extremely pale and with his head bent to one side" (28).

Given the evidence summarized above, Lanza likely succumbed to a massive pulmonary embolus, a myocardial infarction, or a hypertensive cerebral hemorrhage. Of the three, a massive pulmonary embolus is the most likely, given Lanza's sudden death shortly after awakening from twilight sleep. His thrombophlebitis posed a constant threat of pulmonary embolism, which would have increased markedly in the aftermath of his prolonged immobilization when a newly formed blood clot would have been in danger of dislodging from the deep veins of his right leg once he resumed walking. If he did die of a pulmonary embolus, it was not likely his only episode of thromboembolization. During a hospitalization for "double pneumonia" in August 1959, he was diagnosed with a simultaneous pulmonary embolism, although the evidence for such is not known (27).

With regard to a fatal myocardial infarction, Lanza reportedly had an enlarged heart as early as April 1958, an electrocardiogram showing evidence of "myocardial damage" (unconfirmed) in February 1959, and a "minor heart attack" in April 1959. His older son, Damon, claimed that his father had another minor heart attack in August 1959 before succumbing to a third fatal one in October (60). However, the specific criteria used to diagnose these myocardial infarctions, unfortunately, are not known. Lanza's younger son, Marc, died of a heart attack at age 37 in 1991 (66).

Lanza's untreated hypertension (with systolic pressures in the range of 290 mm Hg) also placed him at extreme risk of cerebral hemorrhage. Therefore, it is also possible that he died of a hypertensive cerebral hemorrhage, one possibly precipitated by hCG-induced thyrotoxicosis.

Although Lanza never realized his dream of an operatic career, according to the son of "the great Caruso," Enrico Jr.: "Mario Lanza [nevertheless] performed an invaluable service to opera. Lanza became a household name; thanks to him opera was no longer an art form for an elite group of eggheads, but was acceptable entertainment for all" (67).

Fifty years after his death, Mario Lanza's voice continues to enrapture listeners with "an impressively round velvety center and a brilliant top with ringing B and B flat, and a splendid and secure C" (68). Truly, his was a voice for the ages, silenced too soon by a life of excess for which medicine had yet to discover a cure.

References

1. Cesari A. *Mario Lanza: An American Tragedy*. Fort Worth, TX: Baskerville Publishers, 2004:xvi–xvii.

2. Parsons L. *Los Angeles Times*, Oct. 8, 1959.

3. Op. cit. Cesari, pp. 5, 247–253.

4. Ibid., pp. 8, 9, 11, 13, 15.

5. Ibid., p. 17.

6. Briggs J. *Leonard Bernstein: The Man, His Works, and His Music*. New York: World Publishing Co., 1961.

7. Op. cit. Cesari, p. 21.

8. *New York Times*, Aug. 9, 1942.

9. *Opera News*, Oct. 5, 1942.

10. Op. cit. Cesari, pp. 25–26.

11. Ibid., pp. 28, 31–33, 81–82.

12. Ibid., pp. 40, 41, 287.

13. Ibid., pp. 44, 67, 69, 71.

14. Ibid., pp. 87, 104–105.

15. Ibid., p. 88.

16. Ibid., pp. 103, 111–112.

17. Ibid., pp. 166–167, 173, 177.

18. Ibid., pp. 184–186.

19. Ibid., pp. 203–204.

20. Ibid., pp. 213, 219.

21. Ibid., pp. 221–222, 234.

22. Ibid., pp. 250–251.

23. Ibid., pp. 255–257.

24. Ibid., pp. 261–264.

25. Ibid., p. 266.

26. Ibid., p. 272.

27. Ibid., pp. 276–277.

28. Ibid., pp. 279–283.

29. Callinicos C. *The Mario Lanza Story*. New York: Coward-McCann Inc., 1960.

30. Barlow SE, the Expert Committee. Expert Committee recommendations regarding the prevention, assessment, and treatment of child and adolescent overweight and obesity: summary report. *Pediatrics* 2007;120(Suppl 4):S164–S192.

31. August GP, Caprio S, Fennoy I, et al. Prevention and treatment of pediatric obesity: an Endocrine Society clinical practice guideline based on expert opinion. *J Clin Endocrinol Metab* 2008;93:4576–4599.

32. Beck MA. Influenza and obesity: will vaccines and antivirals protect? *J Infect Dis* 2012;205:172–173.

33. Pi-Sunyer X. The medical risks of obesity. *Postgrad Med* 2009;121:21–33.

34. Flegal KM, Carroll MD, Kit BK, Ogden CL. Prevalence of obesity and trends in the distribution of body mass index among US adults, 199–2010. *JAMA* 2012;307:491–497.

35. Consensus Development Conference Panel. NIH conference. Gastrointestinal surgery for severe obesity. *Ann Intern Med* 1991;115:956–961.

36. Livingston EH. Inadequacy of BMI as an indicator for bariatric surgery. *JAMA* 2012;307:88–89.

37. Li Z, Heber D. Overeating and overweight. Extra calories increase fat mass while protein increases lean mass. *JAMA* 2012;307:86–87.

38. Sjöström L, Narbo K, Sjöström CD, et al.; Swedish Obese Subjects Study. Effects of bariatric surgery on mortality in Swedish obese subjects. *N Engl J Med* 2007;357:741–752.

39. Maciejewski ML, Livingston EH, Arterburn DE. Survival after bariatric surgery among high-risk patients [letter]. *JAMA* 2011;306:1323–1324.

40. Foxcroft L. *Calories & Corsets. A History of Dieting Over 2000 Years*. London: Profile Books, 2011:15.

41. Ibid., pp. 198, 207.

42. Ibid., p. 2.

43. Maciejewski ML, Livingston EH, Smith VA, et al. Survival among high-risk patients after bariatric surgery. *JAMA* 2011;305:2419–2426.

44. Sjöström L, Rissanen A, Andersen T, et al. European Multicentre Orlistat Study Group. Randomised placebo-controlled trial of orlistat for weight loss and prevention of weight regain in obese patients. *Lancet* 1998;352:167–172.

45. Torgerson JS, Hauptman J, Boldrin MN, Sjöström L. XENical in the prevention of diabetes in obese subjects (XENDOS) study: a randomized study of orlistat as an adjunct to lifestyle changes for the prevention of type 2 diabetes in obese patients. *Diabetes Care* 2004;27:155–161.

46. Sjöström L Lindroos AK Peltonen M, et al. Swedish Obese Subjects Study Scientific Group. Lifestyle, diabetes, and cardiovascular risk factors 10 years after bariatric surgery. *N Engl J Med* 2004;351:2683–2693.

47. Després JP, Golay A, Sjöström L; Rimonabant in Obesity-Lipids Study Group. Effects of rimonabant on metabolic risk factors in overweight patients with dyslipidemia. *N Engl J Med* 2005;353:2121–2134.

48. Lee IM, Paffenbarger RS Jr. Change in body weight and longevity. *JAMA* 1992;268:2045–2049.

49. Walker MWG, Wannamethee G, Whincup PH, Shaper AD. Weight change and risk of heart attack in middle-aged British men. *Int J Epidemiol* 1995;24:694–703.

50. Nilsson PM, Nilsson JA, Hedblad B, et al. The enigma of increased non-cancer mortality after weight loss in healthy men who are overweight or obese. *J Intern Med* 2002;252:70–78.

51. Pamuk ER, Williamson DF, Serdula MK, et al. Weight loss and subsequent death in a cohort of U.S. adults. *Ann Intern Med* 1993;119:744–748.

52. Nissen SE, Nicholls SJ, Wolski K, et al., STRADIVARIUS Investigators. Effect of rimonabant on progression of atherosclerosis in patients with abdominal obesity and coronary artery disease: the STRADIVARIUS randomized controlled trial. *JAMA* 2008;299:1547–1560.

53. James WP, Caterson ID, Coutinho W, et al., SCOUT Investigators. Effect of sibutramine on cardiovascular outcomes in overweight and obese subjects. *N Engl J Med* 2010;363:905–917.

54. Petrov DB. Starvation diets as a cause of acquired long QT syndrome [letter]. *Ann Intern Med* 2009;150:501.

55. Op. cit. Foxcroft, p. 200.

56. Cecil RL, Loeb RF, eds. *A Textbook of Medicine*. Philadelphia and London: W. B. Saunders Co., 1959:1188–1198.

57. Ibid., pp. 1620–1630.

58. Ibid., pp. 1342–1344.

59. Ibid., pp. 1283–1291.

60. Lanza D, Dolfi B, Muller M. *Be My Love. A Celebration of Mario Lanza*. Chicago: Bonus Books, Inc., 1999:220–222.

61. ABC 4 Investigation: Pregnancy hormone for weight loss. http://www.abc4. com/news/local/story/ABC-4-Investigation-Pregnancy-hormone-for-weight/ jUZY95Pokou83IRWEU-hrg.cspx (June 3, 2009).

62. Simeons ATW. The action of chorionic gonadotropin in the obese. *Lancet* 1954;267(6845):946–947.

63. Simeons ATW. Chorionic gonadotropin in the obese [letter]. *Lancet* 1962;ii:47–48.

64. Lox C, Canez M, DeLeon F, et al. Hyperestrogenism induced by menotropins alone or in conjunction with leuprolide acetate in in-vitro fertilization cycles: the impact on hemostasis. *Fertil Steril* 1995;63:566–570.

65. Glinoer D. The regulation of thyroid function in pregnancy: pathways of endocrine adaptation from physiology to pathology. *Endocrine Rev* 1997;18:404–414.

66. Op. cit. Cesari, p. 289.

67. Ibid., p. 120.

68. Ibid., p. 72.

13 "Too Busy to Be Sick"

THIS PATIENT WAS no ordinary First Lady. She shattered the traditional mold of the position and refashioned it to fit her talents and to serve as an instrument of social reform. She was the first American chief executive's wife to hold—and lose—a government job and the first to testify before Congress, to address a national party convention, to hold regular press conferences, to write a syndicated daily column, to deliver sponsored radio broadcasts, to earn income on the lecture circuit, and to travel overseas to visit American troops in combat (1).

Her husband was President of the United States during as trying a time as any this nation has yet faced. He lost the use of his legs to polio 16 years after they were married, and had she not been so steadfast and raised her voice so vigorously against her mother-in-law in behalf of full recovery, he could easily have become an invalid (2). Fortunately for the country, she refused to treat him as an invalid and wouldn't allow others to do so. Though confined to a wheelchair for the remainder of his life, he persevered in politics and was elected President in 1932, a decade after becoming paralyzed, and then reelected in 1936, in 1940, and again in 1944. To no small degree, she was the one who made it possible for him to carry on in spite of his disability (3).

When a world war came to dominate her husband's presidency, the patient became his principal advisor on social issues (4), the "eyes and ears" that gathered the grassroots information he needed to understand the people he governed (5). She traveled incessantly for him, performing inspections that were thorough to the extreme. When, for example, she visited a military hospital in the South Pacific during the war, she didn't just shake hands with the chief medical officer, glance into a sunroom, and leave. She went into every ward, stopped at every bed, and spoke to every patient. What was his name? How did he feel? Was there anything he needed? Could she take a message home for him? And when she made a promise, it was a promise kept (6). She saw things the President couldn't see and described them with such poignant understanding that he came to depend greatly on her reports (7).

For two decades during her husband's presidency she was indefatigable as a social activist. She fought for racial equality—in the military as well as on the home front; for workers' rights and assistance for the poor and unemployed; for female employment and industry-sponsored day-care programs; for educational support for returning veterans through the GI Bill; for repeal of her husband's decision to incarcerate thousands of West Coast Japanese-Americans in the interest of national security; for America to open its doors to refugees of the Holocaust; for financial assistance to war-ravaged Europe (8); and for creation of the United Nations (9). She also lobbied hard for civilian conscription, reasoning that whereas the draft was vital to winning the world war, a wider form of national service involving every citizen was needed to ensure that the country emerged from the war worthy of the many lives that had been sacrificed (10, 11).

She pushed her husband hard on such issues, some said "too hard at the end of the day, when he was tired and needed to relax." More often than not, to the nation's benefit, he came around to her way of thinking (12).

Because of such dedication and influence, she became "the most admired person in the world" (13), "a cabinet minister without portfolio" (14), and "the most influential woman of her time" (14). However, there were also many who dismissed her as a "busybody," a "meddler," and a "gab," for not being a systematic thinker, unable to focus or set priorities, and victimized by overly generous impulses that drove her to intervene on behalf of anyone in trouble, whether his or her complaints were justified or not (12). They considered her a dreamer for believing that either war or poverty could ever be eliminated. She talked too damned much and needed to be muzzled. She needed to stop going around the country stirring up colored people, telling them they were as good as white people. She ought to stay home, where a wife belongs, they complained, instead of getting her nose into the government's business and acting as if the people had elected her President (15). Never once did the President bend to such criticism to curb the generous idealism and humanitarian impulses that motivated her social activism (12).

When her husband had a massive stroke and died in March 1945, just as the war with the Axis powers was about to be won, the patient felt that she had done all she could do (16). "The story is over," she said (17). However, the story was far from over. In December 1945, President Truman asked her to serve as a member of the

American delegation to the first meeting of the United Nations General Assembly. She accepted, though with trepidation given her lack of experience in foreign affairs. Then, for nearly two decades, she served on Committee Three of the United Nations as America's foremost champion of universal human rights. Although the only woman in the U.S. delegation, she was elected chairperson by acclamation of the U.N. Human Rights Commission. And when her strength began to ebb as she approached her eighth decade, she took on additional assignments, this time for President Kennedy, as a member of the Advisory Council of the Peace Corps (18).

The patient came from a storied, if troubled, American family. Teddy Roosevelt was her uncle. Unfortunately, Teddy's brother, her father, inherited neither the drive nor the strength of character of his famous sibling. Though warm and affectionate while sober, he was ruled by alcohol. After years of heavy drinking, he developed delirium tremens and died at the age of 34, when the patient was 8. Many years later, alcohol also claimed the life of a younger brother. Her only other sibling, another brother, died of diphtheria at the age of 4 (19).

The patient's mother was a debutante of such great beauty that the poet Robert Browning is said to have asked to be allowed to sit and gaze at her while she had her portrait painted (20). By comparison, the patient was plain and ungainly, even more so as a child because of a brace she had to wear for several years for curvature of the spine. Her self-absorbed and bitterly disappointed mother tried to compensate for her daughter's lack of beauty by teaching her excellent manners, which only made the child more keenly aware of her shortcomings (21). Her mother contracted diphtheria and died the same year as the patient's father (19).

A lesser child's spirit would have been broken by such maternal disaffection, but not this child's. In time, she came to believe that "no one can make you feel inferior without your consent" (22). Even so, the legacy of repeated loss as a child left her forever starved for love and prone to recurring depression. It also produced resilient strength—strength to do things she thought she could not do: dealing with a dominating mother-in-law, her husband's infidelity and death, the death of a 20-month-old child, the disappointing careers and broken marriages of her five surviving children, and her many years of swimming against the tide of prejudice and fear (23).

Prior to her terminal illness, the patient's health had been consistently excellent. In May 1953, she entered Columbia-Presbyterian Hospital for the first time, because of pain in her left hand. "An operation on the lower left forearm showed chronic inflammation of the tendon sheath. She made a complete recovery" (24). Otherwise, she rarely even contracted a cold, and once boasted she had never had a headache. Her attitude toward illness was that "if she ignored anything wrong with anyone, it wouldn't exist" (25). She simply "wasn't interested in physiology"

(26). She believed that iron will and courage could conquer any illness (42). Though deeply compassionate, she had no patience for illness—hers or anyone else's (27)—and so she was totally unprepared for the pernicious disorder that crept into her life in early 1960.

She was 75 and campaigning for John F. Kennedy with stump speeches in a half-dozen states from California to New York to West Virginia. The illness began with fatigue she thought was due to a virus she had picked up. At first she expected it to go away and ignored it. However, gradually she became so weary she began falling asleep on her feet and had to be helped to a chair before toppling over. Reluctantly, she consulted her personal physician, Dr. A. David Gurewitsch (28).

The series of blood tests Gurewitsch ordered in April 1960 revealed mild anemia, with a hemoglobin level of 10.3 gm% (normal = 12–16 gm%) and a slightly low white blood cell count of 4,450 per cu mm (normal = 5,000–10,000 per cu mm). Gurewitsch referred her to a hematologist for a bone marrow aspiration, which revealed *hyper*cellularity with an excess number of immature white blood cells (i.e., 18 percent myeloblasts). Although the marrow looked suspicious for an early stage of leukemia, the patient's doctors diagnosed "aplastic anemia"—a bone marrow that was losing its capacity to manufacture blood (29). The condition, they explained, was incurable, its cause unknown. Transfusions could bring temporary relief, but sooner or later, her marrow would break down completely and internal hemorrhaging would result (28). Undaunted by the grim prognosis, the patient resumed her journeys around the globe, stating that she wanted nothing more of doctors or their tests (29). She was, she said, "too busy to be sick" (30).

In January 1961, the patient was invited to sit in the presidential box at Kennedy's inauguration but declined, preferring to fend off the icy cold in the stand below rather than sit next to "Old Joe," the president's father. Two months later she developed soreness and swelling of her legs, which she attributed to a bout of influenza. Her son later claimed that the cause was phlebitis and that "the experience drove her to have a new will drawn" (28).

In September 1961, she was admitted to Columbia-Presbyterian Hospital after 2 days of vaginal bleeding for the first time since her menopause at age 50. "She had been receiving irregular treatment for the previous several months with Premarin (a female sex hormone preparation)... to see if it would have a beneficial affect [sic] on her poorly functioning bone marrow" (24). The Premarin had caused her uterus to hypertrophy and bleed. Following curettage, she "left the hospital...feeling as well as she did before" (24). When admitted to the hospital, her hemoglobin had dropped two points to 8.2 gm%. More ominous were her low white blood cell count of 1500 per cu mm (with 79 percent lymphocytes), her platelet count of 79,000 per cu mm (normal = 200,000–500,000), and her elevated erythrocyte sedimentation rate (ESR, a marker of inflammation) of 50 mm per hr (normal ≤20 mm per hr). A repeat bone marrow aspiration revealed *hypo*cellularity with only 5 percent immature white blood cells (myeloblasts). Just as her physicians had predicted, her marrow was shutting down, losing its capacity to produce any of the blood elements. When transfused with two units of blood to raise her low hemoglobin level, she developed high fever and chills—her first of many transfusion reactions. A chest x-ray performed on September 5 "revealed large calcified nodes in both hilar areas [the sites at which nerves and vessels enter and leave the lungs], more marked on the left." The fever abated quickly, and after 3 days in the hospital, the patient was sent home (31).

When visited by her son and daughter-in-law shortly after Christmas, the patient looked ill and very old. Her shoulders were stooped, her cheeks puffy (28).

In February 1962, she traveled abroad for the last time, visiting Israel and Switzerland. Then, in April, Gurewitsch, in consultation with Columbia-Presbyterian hematologist Dr. George Hyman, made what turned out to be a crucial decision. In view of a hemoglobin level that had fallen to 7.9 gm%, a white blood count of only 1,800 per cu mm, a platelet count of 87,000 per cu mm, and frequent bruising, they decided to begin treatment with 20 mg prednisone, given in 5-mg doses four times a day, hoping the drug would stimulate production of her red blood cells and platelets. They knew that such high doses of corticosteroid drugs like prednisone, especially when given in divided doses throughout the day, suppress the body's ability to fight certain infections (in particular tuberculosis) but believed that the risk was worth the potential benefit of alleviating the aplastic anemia. The daily dose of prednisone was reduced to 15 mg on July 9, then 12.5 mg on July 16, and 10 mg thereafter (31).

The patient's illness was kept secret from the public. As the 1962 campaign gained steam, she felt obligated to do her bit once again for the Committee for Democratic Voters. Though she was failing fast, she agreed to speak at an open-air rally (28).

She needed help getting out of the car when she arrived. "I had to come; I was expected," she explained to the girl waiting for her with a bouquet. As she climbed the steps to the platform on which she was to speak, a group of teenagers wearing lapel buttons of the newly formed Conservative Party began chanting: "Communist, go back to Russia!" She ignored them and spoke for 15 minutes. When she had finished and was making her way through the audience shaking every hand in reach, the chanting resumed. As she slumped into the seat of the car that was to take her away, she murmured for the first time: "I don't feel very well" (28).

Despite the prednisone, the patient continued to require periodic transfusions. By this time, her normally steady hand wavered so that her letters were all but illegible. She told her children that the one way left for her to help them was to die so that they could receive their inheritance (28).

In July, her illness entered a new phase with the onset of "low grade fever with frequent night sweats and a mild cough" (24). In early August, she developed 4 days of fever to 105°F (40.5°C) following a transfusion. The fever abated but only temporarily. She could no longer count on a day when chills or fever would not force her to rest. Rather than cancel one of the many appearances that were still being demanded of her, she had her assistant call one of her children to "pinch-hit," selling bonds for Israel, raising funds for her charities and other selfless projects. She told her children that she wanted her eyes to go to an eye bank for the blind, and that she wished to be buried in a simple oak coffin, covered not with flowers but with branches of evergreen from the Val-Kill woods in which her beloved cottage stood. She requested further that her wrists be opened for fear of being buried alive (28).

The patient was admitted again to the Columbia-Presbyterian Medical Center in an effort to determine the cause of her fever. An admission note dated August 4, 1962, by Dr. Alfred Gellhorn, a cancer specialist, described several days of fever, chills, and night sweats, along with several weeks of a dry cough. The patient's hemoglobin level was now 7.5 gm%, her white blood count a mere 200 per cu mm (with 69 percent polymorphonuclear leukocytes and 31 percent lymphocytes), and her platelet count 83,000 per cu mm. Her ESR had risen sharply to 128 mm per hr. Her chest x-ray "revealed questionable widening of the superior mediastinum and the bilateral hilar adenopathy," thought to be due to contact with tuberculosis in 1919 when she had been told that she had had a touch of pleurisy (31). "The prednisone, which had been decreased by the patient in late July to 2.5 mg daily, was increased to 30 mg daily in view of the fever... Because of bright red rectal bleeding, a dilatation of the anal sphincter was performed and an excision of hypertrophied anal papillae with cauterization of petechial areas of bleeding was performed... with good results" (31).

Gurewitsch worried that the long-dormant focus of suspected tuberculosis had reactivated (31). "But when he later took it up with the drs. Conference and said it might be tb of the bone marrow, they all scoffed at him—it's a typical a-leukemic, leukemia, they said the blood specialists" (32).

Tuberculosis, also known as *consumption*, *phthisis*, and *the wasting disease*, has probably always been with us. Paleopathological evidence indicates that it was prevalent in Egypt as early as 3700 BCE and in Europe as far back as 2500 to 1500 BCE. It is the subject of a hymn in the *Riga Veda*, a sacred text of India dating from 2500 BCE (33) and has been detected in the mummified remains of Native Americans traced to the first millennium, confirming its existence in the New World prior to the arrival of Columbus (34). Before the advent of effective antituberculosis drugs, it was so widespread and so lethal it came to be known as *the great white plague* (35).

Until the work of French surgeon Jean-Antoine Villemin and German general practitioner Robert Koch, the cause of tuberculosis was unknown. Many believed it was inherited, others that it was a form of cancer (36). Although regarded as nothing short of a death sentence, for a time the disease was considered a fashionable way to die. "I look pale," Lord Byron mused in 1828. "I should like to die of consumption...the ladies would say 'Look at that poor Byron, how interesting he looks in dying'" (37).

As the Industrial Revolution gathered steam, the urban poor, malnourished and overcrowded, became the principal target of tuberculosis. The infection became a disease of the masses, no longer an expression of a refined character but a disorder indicative of weakness, ignorance, and immorality. Koch dispelled any lingering notion that it reflected artistic or spiritual virtue by demonstrating that the disease was an infection, one caused by a microbe, *Mycobacterium tuberculosis*, that is inhaled into the lungs inside droplets coughed up by a sick contact. Eventually, it begins to breed in the lungs, causing inflammatory cells to migrate to sites of infection and wall the bacteria off, creating inflammatory nodules called "tubercles" (37). In over 90 percent of patients, the infection is permanently arrested as a result of the action of inflammatory cells. Of those patients who are unable to contain the infection, most develop a progressively destructive process of the uppermost areas of the lungs within 2 years of the initial infection, when for as-yet-unclear reasons, bacteria escape from the tubercles in which they had been confined. Many fewer develop a disseminated form of the infection, in which mycobacteria released into the bloodstream spread to tissues throughout the body. Corticosteroid drugs like prednisone, AIDS, and certain cancers and their treatments predispose persons to active tuberculosis by inhibiting inflammatory cells' ability to contain *M. tuberculosis* within tubercles (38).

Fortunately for mankind, 1943 marked a turning point in the struggle against tuberculosis. A New Jersey poultry farmer upset over a strange infection his chickens seemed to be catching from barnyard dirt took the birds to the Rutgers University laboratory of Dr. Selman Waksman. In work for which he later received the Nobel Prize, Waksman isolated a peculiar bacterium, *Streptomyces griseus*, from the barnyard soil, then discovered that the bacterium produced an antibiotic, *streptomycin*, that inhibited the growth of a wide variety of bacteria, including *M. tuberculosis*. This first antituberculosis drug was followed by the rediscovery of isoniazid (INH) in 1952. A third antituberculosis drug, para-aminosalicylic acid (PAS), also became available in the early 1950s (37). Many others followed. So successful were they in combating tuberculosis that by 1970, few American physicians were aware that the infection still posed a threat to certain segments of the population (39). In 1984, the United States recorded its lowest incidence of the infection in history (37).

In 1985, everything changed with the advent of the AIDS epidemic. Once thought destined for extinction, tuberculosis returned in force, not just in the form of a reemerging epidemic, but one fueled by virulent drug-resistant strains of the bacterium. Despite being declared a global emergency by the World Health Organization in 1995, against which numerous major initiatives have since been directed, the global burden of tuberculosis is higher today than at any other time in history. It remains one of the most important causes of death from infection, with 8 million new cases occurring annually worldwide and 1.45 million tuberculosis-related deaths (40).

During the patient's hospitalization in August 1962, she was treated for 4 days with penicillin and streptomycin for a possible pyogenic bacterial infection (not tuberculosis) while her doctors awaited the results of blood cultures, all of which were negative. Her bone marrow was unchanged (31). She was intermittently confused and angry over her inability to force herself back to health, and then because she was not allowed to die. The endless fussing over blood tests and temperature, not to mention her bone marrow, all seemed so senseless. No sooner was she able to leave her bed than she demanded to be taken home. She was expected at Campobello Island in Canada for the dedication of a memorial bridge to her husband and was determined to attend (28).

On August 10, she was discharged from the hospital without an explanation for her fever. Her physicians had been tapering her prednisone dose, but then, suspecting that the aplastic anemia itself was responsible for the fever, they increased the dose to 25 mg daily (31).

During much of the time traveling to and from Campobello, the patient was only dimly aware of her surroundings. She begged Dr. Gurewitsch, not for the first time, to hasten her exit. Instead, he readmitted her to the hospital on September 26 for additional tests (28). Desperately ill and not wanting anyone else to see her so low, she "asked just one person outside the immediate family to visit her sick room...Adlai Stevenson" (24).

During this admission she had persistent fever with an odd pattern of temperature peaks occurring in the morning rather than the usual afternoon/early evening peaks (Fig. 13.1) (31). She was deathly pale, covered with bruises, and passing black tarry stools indicative of intestinal hemorrhaging. Her face was strangely rounded in appearance, and she had ulcers in her mouth caused by a fungal infection (candidiasis), both commonly seen in patients on prolonged prednisone therapy. Her hemoglobin level was 6.2 gm%, her white blood cell count

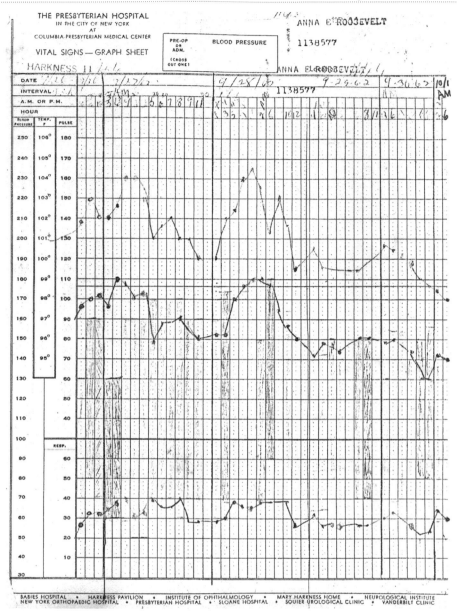

FIGURE 13.1 The patient's Presbyterian Hospital Vital Signs-Graph Sheet during her September 1962 admission. The temperature curve (*top*) is odd to the extent that while febrile, the patient's peak temperatures (on September 27 and 28) occur in the morning rather than the late afternoon/early evening, when such peaks typically occur.

900 per cu mm (with 17 percent myeloblasts and one nucleated red blood cell). She needed oxygen to relieve her shortness of breath and had had so many past injections and blood samples taken that the nurses had difficulty finding a vein in which to administer intravenous fluids (28). Her chest x-ray had changed: it now "presented a generalized ill-defined nodularity which had not been present 7 days previously on an outside study" (31).

Given the patient's persistent fever and chills along with the nodular pulmonary infiltrate, a "group consultation" held on September 27 finally decided that tuberculosis needed to be ruled out—not pulmonary tuberculosis but *miliary* tuberculosis, a disseminated form of the infection in which the organism spreads via the bloodstream throughout the body, creating tiny foci of infection the size of millet seeds in nearly every organ. The procedure chosen to rule out miliary tuberculosis was yet another bone marrow examination—not an aspiration this time, but a biopsy with a larger bore Vim-Silverman needle. Microscopic examination of the biopsy specimen revealed "normal cellularity but again failed to show any definite evidence of leukemia...or tuberculous granulomata" (31). Nevertheless, because *M. tuberculosis* is difficult to identify microscopically in patients with disseminated tuberculosis, the patient's team of physicians decided to treat her empirically with streptomycin and INH while awaiting the results of the bone marrow culture. In view of her intestinal bleeding and an extremely low platelet count, they added alternate-day injections of testosterone to her daily prednisone (31).

The patient's fever resolved several days after initiation of therapy with the two antituberculosis drugs. However, within another few days it returned, reaching 105°F (40.5°C) on October 12. She continued to bleed per rectum and to suffer an allergic reaction each time she received a blood transfusion. Two barium enemas in search of a cause for her intestinal bleeding revealed nothing of importance (31).

Determined to die, with or without the help of her physicians, the patient began spitting out pills or hiding them under her tongue. Nothing the doctors did made sense to her. She refused further testing and demanded to go home. Finally, having performed "all of the diagnostic measures that could be done...her attending physicians felt that they could accede to her request to return to her home" (31). On October 18, 1962, 4 days after U-2 reconnaissance revealed Soviet missiles being installed in Cuba, and 7 days after her 78th birthday, she was carried out of the hospital on a stretcher (28). Her discharge medications included digitoxin and Mercuhydrin for trace ankle edema, prednisone (15 mg every 6 hours), Gelusil, isoniazid, colimycin (intramuscular), streptomycin (intramuscular), and penicillin (intramuscular) (31).

Eight days later, the results of the bone marrow culture arrived. *M. tuberculosis* was growing in the culture tubes that had been inoculated with the patient's marrow. Dr. Gurewitsch was ecstatic: not only had his suspicion been confirmed, but he now had a curable disease to treat. Though his patient's hemoglobin had dropped to 3.6 gm% and her platelets to only 30,000 per cu mm (31), he assured her that her chances for survival "had gone up by 5000%" (29).

The patient's family was not impressed. Their mother's suffering, they argued, had gone on long enough (29). Undeterred, Dr. Gurewitsch doubled the dose of INH and continued transfusing his patient at her home with blood that had been vigorously washed to prevent further allergic reactions. He also had her trachea suctioned repeatedly to clear it of secretions and a catheter placed into her bladder to monitor her urinary output while hoping for a miracle that was not to be (31).

Years later Gurewitsch reflected upon the suffering he and his colleagues had inflicted upon their helpless patient with their endless tests and ineffectual treatments. "He had not done well by Mrs. R. toward the end, he said. She had told him that if her illness flared up again and fatally that she did not want to linger on and expected him to save her from the protracted, helpless, dragging out of suffering. But he could not do it, he said. When the time came, his duty as a doctor prevented him" (24).

"In spite of these measures, the patient became increasingly somnolent and...[had] increasing difficulty with oral secretions...with coughing spells...The blood pressure fell and the pulse became thready and weak...[The patient] rallied slightly but she was essentially comatose from November 5 until the late afternoon of November 7, when she had marked difficulty with oral secretions, relieved by oral and nasal suction and then by tracheal suction by Dr. Leonard Brand of the Anesthesia Department. Approximately ten minutes after relief of this last episode, [the patient] became cyanotic, the heart failed, and shortly thereafter respiration ceased. Attempts at closed chest resuscitation with mouth-to-mouth breathing, and the use of intracardiac adrenalin were not successful" (31).

At 6:15 p.m. on November 7, 1962, Dr. Gurewitsch's patient's suffering ended. On that day, Anna Eleanor Roosevelt (Fig. 13.2), "trooper to the last" (41), died 3 days after having suffered a massive stroke (32). When the terms of her will were announced, only $150,000 remained to be distributed—just a small fraction of the fortune she had amassed over the years. Most of her earnings she had given to charity and other good causes. Money, she believed, was something to be given to those with needs greater than her own (28).

An autopsy confirmed the presence of both "aplastic anemia" and disseminated tuberculosis (Fig. 13.3) (31). Myriad clusters of *M. tuberculosis* were found in Roosevelt's lungs, liver, spleen, kidneys, and bone marrow. Moreover, there were none of the inflammatory granulomas (tubercles) one expects to see in a patient struggling to fend off such an infection. Roosevelt's organs contained

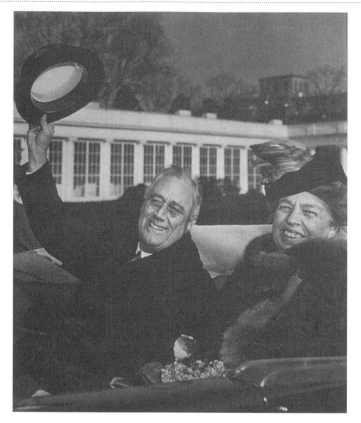

FIGURE 13.2 Eleanor Roosevelt with Franklin D. Roosevelt in the back seat of an open limousine arriving at the White House following her husband's inauguration as President in 1941.

only vast numbers of bacteria and dead tissue. The destruction of her organs by *M. tuberculosis* was so extensive that the pathologist labeled her disorder *disseminated tuberculosis acutissima* rather than "miliary tuberculosis," which he felt would not adequately convey the magnitude of the damage caused by the infection. Roosevelt's physicians speculated that her immune-compromised state—due to both her bone marrow failure and prednisone therapy—had allowed a long-dormant focus of tuberculosis to escape from the granuloma in which it had been confined since 1919, enter the bloodstream, and disseminate throughout her body. Because of the near-total absence of an immune response to the infection, she was unable to mount the characteristic pulmonary nodules typically seen in patients with miliary tuberculosis (29, 31).

When the results of susceptibility tests performed on the *M. tuberculosis* isolated from Roosevelt's marrow returned, her physicians were confronted with perhaps the greatest shock of all. In spite of the fact that the particular strain responsible for her disseminated tuberculosis was thought to have been contracted in 1919,

ANNE ELEANOR ROOSEVELT   AGE: 78   AUTOPSY 20,993

WARD: Patient Expired at Home   HISTORY 1138577

ADMISSION: Many Previous Admissions   X-RAY   1138577

DIED: 11/7/62   at 6:15 P.M.

AUTOPSY: 11/7/62   DRS. SPIRO AND WIENER

FINAL ANATOMIC DIAGNOSES

APLASTIC ANEMIA, (Steroid treated), with
    hypocellular bone marrow and petechial
    hemorrhages of skin
    Fibrocalcific tuberculosis (old) involving
      both pulmonary apices and hilar lymph nodes
    Disseminated tuberculosis acutissima (treated)
      involving lungs, liver, spleen, kidneys,
      hilar lymph nodes and left temporal lobe
    Active duodenal ulcer, steroid induced

SECONDARY DIAGNOSES
    Generalized arteriosclerosis, slight
    Hydronephrosis and hydroureter, slight, right
    Superficial cystitis (catheter)
    Diverticulae, jejunal, multiple
    Nabothian cysts
    Cystic dilatation of endometrial glands

FIGURE 13.3 Eleanor Roosevelt's final anatomical diagnoses as they appear on her actual autopsy report (31).

nearly 40 years before the advent of the two drugs with which she was treated, her isolate was resistant to both streptomycin and INH (Fig. 13.3). Her physicians were mystified (29, 31).

Ask the average present-day physician with any knowledge of Eleanor Roosevelt what she died of, and chances are the answer will be something like "miliary tuberculosis masquerading as aplastic anemia" or "miliary tuberculosis misdiagnosed as leukemia"... "a curable disease mishandled by physicians at one of the country's most prestigious hospitals" (30). But was Roosevelt's case mismanaged by physicians at Columbia-Presbyterian Hospital? Did she have disseminated tuberculosis all along, which masqueraded as aplastic anemia, or did she have some other blood disorder, like leukemia, that looked like aplastic anemia but wasn't and should have been treated differently? Was prednisone indicated; should it have been discontinued once it was clear it wasn't alleviating her "aplastic anemia;" did it convert a dormant focus of tuberculosis into a raging disseminated infection? Why was her strain of *M. tuberculosis* resistant to streptomycin and INH if it had originated decades before either drug was around?

"Aplastic anemia" (42–44) is one of several bone marrow failure syndromes in which the precursor cells that constitute the marrow—cells responsible for producing red blood cells, white blood cells, and platelets—progressively disappear and are replaced by fat. Most cases of the disorder are "idiopathic"—that is, their cause is unknown. The hallmark of the disorder is a *hypo*cellular marrow. A *hyper*cellular marrow with an increased number of immature white blood cells (myeloblasts), as was reported for Roosevelt's initial aspirate, would be inconsistent with aplastic anemia, even in its early stage.

An enormous literature dating back nearly a century incriminated numerous drugs and chemicals as causes of aplastic anemia (45). The antibiotic chloramphenicol (which Roosevelt did receive, but apparently only once during her final hospitalization in 1962 (31)), in particular, was long believed to cause the disorder. However, on critical review, the data supporting such associations are inconclusive, and current evidence favors an immunological basis for marrow failure in nearly all cases. Nevertheless, the fundamental question of why a patient's immune system begins to attack her bone marrow continues to be a mystery. The cause is unknown . . . *idiopathic* (42).

Prior to the advent of hematopoietic stem-cell transplantation (transplantation of marrow precursor cells) and modern immune-suppressive drug therapy, the disorder was nearly always fatal. In the 1960s, prednisone was the immune-suppressive drug of choice and would have been a reasonable treatment for Roosevelt's aplastic anemia, if in fact that was what she had.

Myelodysplastic syndrome (MDS) (46, 47) can also cause the marrow to fail. However, unlike aplastic anemia, it is malignant disorder (i.e., a cancer), actually a group of cancers involving one or more of the cell lines populating the marrow. Its various subtypes display striking clinical, pathological, and genetic heterogeneity and variable likelihood of progressing to full-blown leukemia. It is more common than aplastic anemia. In fact, it is one of the most common hematological cancers of the elderly in Western countries and a more likely cause of Roosevelt's blood disorder than aplastic anemia. In contrast to aplastic anemia, it typically presents with a *hyper*cellular marrow accompanied by low numbers of circulating red blood cells, white blood cells, and/or platelets. This paradox—high numbers of precursor cells in the marrow with low numbers of mature blood elements in the bloodstream—reflects the death of the former before they can be released into the periphery.

In most cases of MDS, the marrow is persistently hypercellular. However, in some 20 percent of cases, it becomes hypocellular over time, much as it did in Eleanor Roosevelt. Old age, low white blood cell and platelet counts, anemia, the need for transfusions, and increased numbers of myeloblasts in the marrow, all of which applied to Roosevelt, are associated with a poor prognosis. Results of bone marrow chromosome analyses are also predictive, but such analyses were not yet available at that time.

The distinction between aplastic anemia and MDS, a condition not recognized until a decade or so after Roosevelt's death, is not merely academic. MDS generally does not respond well to immune-suppressive drugs such as prednisone. The most effective treatment currently available is hematopoietic stem-cell transplantation. Drugs effective in treating MDS, notably the demethylating agents azacitidine and decitabine, have become available only in the last decade. Patients are also supported with periodic red blood cell transfusions for symptomatic anemia, platelet transfusions for bleeding, and judicious use of hematopoietic cytokines (marrow stimulants). Just a few patients stabilize temporarily on prednisone (48).

Roosevelt's physicians were justified in giving her a trial of prednisone to see if it would alleviate, or at least stabilize, her "aplastic anemia." However, after several weeks of such therapy, when it had become clear that prednisone was not producing the desired effect, perhaps they should have stopped administering the drug, given its potent immune-suppressive effect. This is not to say that they mismanaged the case, either according to standards of their day or for that matter according to modern standards. All too often, even today, rather than discontinue a drug that is not working, physicians simply add another or, as in the case of Roosevelt, increase the dose of the ineffective drug in the mistaken belief that if a drug is indicated for a particular disorder, it should be continued even if not producing the desired effect, as long as it is not causing problems of its own.

Rarely, if ever, does aplastic anemia or MDS cause fever or an elevated ESR. These are usually due to a pyogenic bacterial infection (infections caused by "typical" bacteria, such as the pneumococcus, intestinal bacteria like *Escherichia coli*, and such) owing to the low number of circulating white blood cells (polymorphonuclear leukocytes) in such patients. Mononuclear leukocytes, the inflammatory cells principally responsible for defense against "atypical" microorganisms, such as *M. tuberculosis*, generally are not impaired in patients with aplastic anemia or MDS. Therefore, tuberculosis is not a particular problem in such patients unless they are treated with medications such as prednisone, which inhibit mononuclear leukocyte function.

It has been known since the early 1960s that when tuberculosis invades the bone marrow, it can radically alter the production of blood cells as well as platelets (49–51). Sometimes it stimulates the marrow, causing it to become hypercellular and release large numbers of white blood cells into the bloodstream, a phenomenon known as a "leukemoid (i.e., leukemia-like) reaction." At other times, it suppresses the marrow, causing it to become hypocellular and produce a picture indistinguishable from aplastic anemia. This being the case, could disseminated tuberculosis alone have been responsible for Roosevelt's hematological disorder and death? Did she have one disease all along, miliary tuberculosis, rather than tuberculosis superimposed on aplastic anemia or MDS? Was prednisone the last drug that she should have received?

Several factors make the "tuberculosis all along" scenario unlikely, the most compelling of which is that Roosevelt did well clinically for more than 2 years (April 1960 to July 1962) after the onset of her hematological disorder. Even given the fact that she had intermittent fevers during this time, 2 years of stable, low-grade, disseminated tuberculosis would be unprecedented. In addition, recent highly sophisticated studies using a nested polymerase chain reaction (N-PCR) assay failed to detect *M. tuberculosis* DNA in bone marrow biopsy samples taken from any of 30 patients with idiopathic aplastic anemia (52). Finally, no patient with tuberculosis and aplastic anemia has ever been reported to recover with antituberculosis therapy alone (53), suggesting that, contrary to earlier reports, tuberculosis is not a cause of aplastic anemia but a complication or, for that matter, a cause of MDS, nor is there a basis for considering tuberculosis a treatable cause of either disorder.

Thus, Roosevelt's tuberculosis was almost certainly superimposed on her hematological disorder, but when did the infection begin? Should it have been diagnosed sooner? Dr. Gurewitsch certainly thought so. He told colleagues: "We could have had the same diagnosis a year ago...she could have been saved. It was left to me to make the diagnosis...Others should have made it, especially the hematologist. The dirty linen will come out!" (29).

There can be little doubt that Roosevelt's tuberculosis was already advancing rapidly in July 1962, when she presented with fever and an ESR of 128 mm per hr, and that the infection should have been considered and, perhaps, diagnosed at that time. By September, she was exhibiting *typhus inversus*, reversal of the usual diurnal pattern of fever with highest temperature elevations in the morning hours rather than during the late afternoon/early evening, an unusual fever pattern sometimes seen in patients with miliary tuberculosis (54). However, disseminated tuberculosis is an elusive disorder. The diagnosis is especially difficult to make in elderly patients like Roosevelt, who are receiving immune-suppressive drugs, which tend to mask classic features of the disorder, such as fever, night sweats, and nodular pulmonary infiltrates. When J. Burns Amberson, chief of the legendary Bellevue chest service and New York City's foremost expert on tuberculosis, was shown Roosevelt's chest x-ray on October 2, 1962, he opined that the nodules present were too irregular and had arisen too quickly to have been due to tuberculosis (29). Even in classic cases of the infection, symptoms such as fever, weight loss, and malaise are nonspecific, and physical findings are minimal. Although it is easy in retrospect to criticize clinicians for missing the diagnosis, even today, many continue to be embarrassed by overlooking the disorder in patients like Roosevelt (55–57).

Ultimately, the question is not so much whether Roosevelt's tuberculosis should have been diagnosed sooner, which *in retrospect* it should have, but whether diagnosing it earlier would have made a difference. Prior to the advent of modern immune-suppressive drugs and stem-cell transplantation, little could be done for patients with either aplastic anemia or MDS: both disorders were nearly invariably fatal in the 1960s. Therefore, if Roosevelt's tuberculosis had been diagnosed earlier and eradicated, she might have lived longer, but not likely much longer. Unfortunately, the strain of *M. tuberculosis* with which she was infected appears to have been resistant to the two principal antituberculosis drugs available at that time. Although an earlier diagnosis of the infection might have induced her physicians to discontinue the prednisone that was inhibiting her natural resistance to *M. tuberculosis*, they had no other effective treatment to offer.

How Roosevelt's strain of *M. tuberculosis* happened to be resistant to both streptomycin and INH is a final mystery. If the source of her disseminated infection was a walled-off collection of bacteria deposited in her lung during a 1919 episode of tuberculous pleurisy, the strain responsible for both the original infection and her subsequent attack of miliary tuberculosis was antituberculosis drug naïve and should have been susceptible to both drugs. Although drug resistance occurs spontaneously in bacteria, the rate at which it does so is extremely low, and it rarely becomes a problem clinically unless resistant strains are given a selective advantage during treatment with drugs that suppress susceptible strains but not the resistant ones. This is a particular problem when antibiotics are used indiscriminately or taken erratically.

In 1962, the incidence of primary drug resistance (i.e., resistance before any treatment is given) among stains of *M. tuberculosis* isolated from patients in the United States was 4.7 percent for streptomycin, 6.0 percent for INH, and 6.1 percent for PAS. Only 0.7 percent of strains were resistant to both streptomycin and INH (58). Drug resistance has increased steadily in the intervening years: strains now exist that are resistant to all currently available drugs, raising concern that we are on the verge of a reemergence of *the white plague* in untreatable form (59). Roosevelt's strain of *M. tuberculosis* might have developed resistance spontaneously to streptomycin and INH in the early 20th century. However, if in fact the susceptibility test results were valid, more likely Roosevelt was infected much later with a resistant strain that had emerged after the introduction of the two drugs, possibly one encountered during her trip to Israel in early 1962, 3 months before her first symptoms of tuberculosis.

To the extent that everything was done that could be done for Roosevelt during the course of her illness, her care was exemplary. And yet, on more critical analysis, in caring for their famous patient, Gurewitsch and his colleagues at the

Columbia-Presbyterian Hospital violated one of the most sacred tenets of medicine, one dating back to the time of Hippocrates—*primum non nocere* ("first, do no harm"). In endeavoring too vigorously through endless tests and treatments to help her overcome her illness, they produced substantially more harm than benefit. Only the transfusions helped by temporarily relieving Roosevelt's symptoms of anemia. The prednisone, continued long after it became apparent that it was not producing the desired effect, brought only *disseminated tuberculosis acutissima*, a bleeding duodenal ulcer, her round ("cushingoid") face and oral candidiasis; the Premarin produced only a hemorrhagic uterus requiring emergency curettage. The numerous intramuscular injections, given in the face of a platelet count of only 30,000 per cu mm, likely did little more than cause painful intramuscular hematomas. And when the time came for their patient to die, Gurewitsch and his colleagues prolonged "the many indignities of being sick and helpless" (32) with washed red cell transfusions, tracheal suctioning, and a urinary catheter, "not to mention umpteen medications" (32). When she did die, and her suffering at last had come to an end, they tried to bring her back to life by performing cardiopulmonary resuscitation (31). Had Eleanor Roosevelt been less famous, perhaps her physicians might have been less concerned with defeating death and more concerned with how they might have prevented her from dying in continuous despair. However, because she was nothing less than the "the First Lady of the World" (24), she was doomed to "dying manifold—without the respite to be dead" (60).

For Eleanor Roosevelt, happiness was not a goal, but a byproduct of doing what she felt in her heart to be right. She fought prejudice and fear with a "tiger's heart wrapped in a woman's hide" (61) and emerged from her famous husband's shadow to achieve greatness of her own. Though she died of a mysterious blood disorder complicated by disseminated tuberculosis, she lives still in the many lives she blessed with her work for peace and human dignity.

References

1. Goodwin DK. *No Ordinary Time. Franklin and Eleanor Roosevelt: the Home Front in World War II*. New York: Simon & Schuster, 1994:110–114.

2. Ibid., p. 568.

3. Rosenman SI. *Working with Roosevelt*. New York: Harper, 1952:364.

4. *U.S. News and World Report*, Dec. 20, 1940, pp. 9–10.

5. Roosevelt E, Brough J. *A Rendezvous with Destiny: The Roosevelts of the White House*. New York: Putnam, 1975:71.

6. Lash JP. *Eleanor and Franklin: the Story of Their Relationship*. New York: Norton, 1971:685.

7. Op. cit. Goodwin, p. 28.

8. Ibid., pp. 82, 88, 98, 102, 161–164, 207, 230, 249, 296–297, 321–323, 331, 364–365, 370–371, 392, 414, 416–418, 423, 430–431, 441–443, 446–447, 454–455, 469, 503, 512, 521–524, 563, 610, 618.

9. Harriman A, Abel D. *Special Envoy to Churchill and Stalin. 1941–1946.* New York: Random House, 1975:222.

10. Roosevelt E. *My Day*, July 11, 1940.

11. *New York Times*, Aug. 28, 1943, p. 3.

12. Op. cit. Goodwin, pp. 628–629.

13. Wills G. *Certain Trumpets: The Call of Leaders.* New York: Simon & Schuster, 1994:62.

14. Hoff-Wilson J, Lightman M, eds. *Without Precedent: The Life and Career of Eleanor Roosevelt.* Bloomington: Indiana University Press, 1984:11.

15. Op. cit. Goodwin, pp. 140, 331, 397.

16. Lash JP. *A World of Love: Eleanor Roosevelt and Her Friends, 1943–1962.* Garden City, NY: Doubleday, 1984:189.

17. *Newsweek*, April 30, 1945, p. 44.

18. Sherman ED. The geriatric profile of Eleanor Roosevelt (1884–1962). *J Am Geriatr Soc* 1983,31:28–33.

19. Op. cit. Goodwin, pp. 91–95, 276.

20. Op. cit. Lash: Eleanor and Franklin, p. 23.

21. Roosevelt E. *This is My Story.* New York: Harper, 1937:11.

22. Roosevelt E. attributed quote, source uncertain.

23. Op. cit. Goodwin, pp. 81, 89, 97–98, 109, 178, 296, 373, 467.

24. FDR Library. Lash Papers. Box 55. Eleanor Roosevelt's Final Illness.

25. Op. cit. Goodwin, p. 541.

26. Asbell B. *Mother and Daughter: Letters of Eleanor and Anna Roosevelt.* New York: Fromm, 1988:177.

27. Op. cit. Goodwin, p. 492.

28. Roosevelt E, Brough J. The last days of Eleanor Roosevelt. *Ladies Home Journal* October 1977:113–226.

29. Lerner BH. Revisiting the death of Eleanor Roosevelt: was the diagnosis of tuberculosis missed? *Int J Tuberc Lung Dis* 2001;5:1080–1085.

30. Lerner BH. *Washington Post*, February 8, 2000:2–10.

31. FDR Library. Anna Roosevelt Halsted Papers. Box 61. Roosevelt, Eleanor Medical Records 1938–1967.

32. FDR Library. Lash Papers. Box 44. Interviews with David Gurewitsch.

33. Kapur V, Whittam TS, Musser JM. Is *Mycobacterium tuberculosis* 15,000 years old? *J Infect Dis* 1994;170:1348–1349.

34. Mackowiak PA, Blos VT, Aguilar M, Buikstra JE. On the origin of American tuberculosis. *Clin Infect Dis* 2005;41:515–518.

35. Otis EO. *The Great White Plague, Tuberculosis.* 2nd ed. New York: Thomas Y. Crowell & Co., 1909.

36. Gröschel DHM. The etiology of tuberculosis: a tribute to Robert Koch on the occasion of the centenary of his discovery of the tubercle bacillus. *ASM News* 1982;48:248–250.

37. Chowder K. How TB survived its own death to confront us again. *Smithsonian* 1992;23:180–194.

38. Fitzgerald DW, Sterling TR, Haas DW. Mycobacterium tuberculosis. In Mandell GL, Bennett JE, Dolin R, eds. *Principles and Practice of Infectious Diseases*, 7th ed. Philadelphia: Churchill Livingstone Elsevier, 2010:3129–3163.

39. Steiner M, Chaves AD, Lyons HA, et al. Primary drug-resistant tuberculosis. Report of an outbreak. *N Engl J Med* 1970;283:1353–1358.

40. Zumla A, Atun R, Maeurer M, et al. Eliminating tuberculosis and tuberculosis-HIV co-disease in the 21st century: key perspectives, controversies, unresolved issues, and needs. *J Infect Dis* 2012;205(Suppl 2):S141–146.

41. Furman B. *Washington By-Line*. New York: Knopf, 1949:314.

42. Young NS, Calado RT, Scheinberg P. Current concepts in the pathophysiology and treatment of aplastic anemia. *Blood* 2006;108:2509–2519.

43. Young NS, Scheinberg P, Calado RT. Aplastic anemia. *Current Opinion in Hematology* 2008;15:162–168.

44. Segel GB, Lichtman MA. Aplastic anemia: acquired and inherited. In Kaushansky K, Lichtman M, Beutler E, et al., eds. *Williams Hematology*, 8th ed. New York: McGraw Hill, 2010:463–483.

45. Girdwood RH. Drug-induced anaemias. *Drugs* 1976;11:394–404.

46. Cazzola M, Della Porta MG, Travaglino E, Malcovati L. Classification and prognostic evaluation of myelodysplastic syndromes. *Semin Oncol* 2011;38:627–634.

47. Lyons RM. Myelodysplastic syndromes: therapy and outlook. *Am J Med* 2012;125(Suppl):S18–23.

48. Young NS, personal communication.

49. Arends A. Blood disease and the so-called generalized non-reactive tuberculosis. *Acta Med Scand* 1950;136:417–428.

50. Evans TS, DeLuca VA Jr, Waters LL. The association of miliary tuberculosis of the bone marrow and pancytopenia. *Ann Intern Med* 1952;37:1044–1052.

51. Ball K, Joules H Pagel W. Acute tuberculous septicaemia with leucopenia. *Br Med J* 1952;2:869–873.

52. Hsu H-C, Lee Y-M, Su W-J, et al. Bone marrow samples from patients with aplastic anemia are not infected with Parvovirus B19 and *Mycobacterium tuberculosis*. *Am J Clin Pathol* 2002;117:36–40.

53. Glasser RM Walker RI, Herion JC. The significance of hematologic abnormalities in patients with tuberculosis. *Arch Intern Med* 1970;125:691–695.

54. Woodward TE. The fever pattern as a diagnostic aid. In Mackowiak PA, ed. *Fever. Basic Mechanisms and Management*, 2nd ed. Philadelphia: Lippincott-Raven, 1997:215–235.

55. Beermann B, Engström J, Hellström, et al. Disseminated tuberculosis in elderly patients. A report on three cases diagnosed intra vitam. *Acta Med Scand* 1971;190:45–48.

56. MacGregor RR. A year's experience with tuberculosis in a private urban teaching hospital in the postsanatorium era. *Am J Med* 1975;58:221–228.

57. Collins MM, Stollerman GH. Disseminated tuberculosis; a presumptive diagnosis. *Hospital Pract* Dec. 15, 1993:53–65.

58. Hobby GL, Johnson PM, Lenert TF, et al. A continuing study of primary drug resistance in tuberculosis in a veteran population within the United States. I. *Am Rev Resp Dis* 1964;89:337–349.

59. Loewenberg S. India reports cases of totally drug-resistant tuberculosis. *Lancet* 2012;379:205.

60. Dickinson E. No. 1013 [c. 1865].

61. Shakespeare W. *Henry VI, I, iv*, 137.

> Diagnosis is a system of more or less accurate guessing, in which the end point achieved is a name. These names applied to disease come to assume the importance of specific entities, whereas they are for the most part no more than insecure and therefore temporary conceptions.
>
> SIR THOMAS LEWIS (1881–1945)

Epilogue

Names applied to diseases—diagnoses—are indeed "temporary conceptions." Those of the past, such as *apoplexy*, *dropsy*, *pulmonic fever*, *intemperance*, *lockjaw*, *old age*, *quinsy*, *rheumatism*, and *white swelling* have given way to *brain attack*, *congestive failure*, *pneumonia*, *ineffective leisure life-style*, *tetanus*, *atherosclerosis*, *pharyngitis*, *gout*, and *anasarca*. Formerly, because physicians had few effective treatments to offer their patients, diagnosis was their paramount, if not only, skill. Today diagnosis is no less important, in that it enables clinicians to select from the myriad available treatments the one most appropriate for the patient at hand. Diagnostic acumen remains the physician's most critical skill...a measure of every doctor's ability and one of the most important components of his or her professional image.

Advances in diagnosis and treatment have benefited mankind in innumerable ways. They have contributed in no small measure to an increase in life expectancy. Patients with what were once terminal disorders, such as tuberculosis, congenital heart disease, and immunodeficiency disorders, now grow old. Many children with cancers are cured. Transplanted vital organs give normal lives back to patients with dead kidneys, livers, and hearts. Cripples have knees and hips replaced and can play tennis again.

Nevertheless, many remain for whom contemporary diagnoses and treatments do little to relieve their suffering or extend their lives. Their plight is exemplified by Tutankhamun, with his multiple congenital abnormalities, the Buddha's super-annuated body, Darwin's intractable "gastric flatus," and Lenin's calcified cerebral vessels. As contemporary patients, each of these giants of the past would have his disorder accorded a name. But, in the words of Benjamin Franklin: "what signifies knowing the name, if you know not the nature of things?" What good is a diagnosis, even the most up-to-date diagnosis, if it does not benefit the patient? Though the physicians who attended Tutankhamun, the Buddha, Darwin, and Lenin had different names for their patients' disorders and different treatments, these were no less informative or effective than those that might be applied to the same patients today. Medicine has come a long way since these famous patients suffered with their mysterious disorders—but for many of today's patients, not yet far enough.

About the Author

Philip A. Mackowiak, MD, MBA, MACP, is Professor and Vice Chairman of the Department of Medicine of the University of Maryland School of Medicine and Chief of the Medical Care Clinical Center of the VA Maryland Health Care System. A graduate of Bucknell University (BS in Biology), the University of Maryland (MD), and the Johns Hopkins University (MBA), he began his career in academic medicine as an Epidemic Intelligence Officer with the Centers for Disease Control in the early 1970s. In 1975, he joined the faculty of the University of Texas Southwestern Medical School in Dallas, where he rose to the rank of Professor of Medicine before returning to the University of Maryland School of Medicine in 1988. He has published more than 150 peer-reviewed articles, editorials, and book chapters on a variety of medical topics, in addition to *Fever: Basic Mechanisms and Management*, the first comprehensive monograph on the diagnosis, prognosis, and treatment of fever since one published by Wunderlich in 1868.

For nearly two decades, Dr. Mackowiak has hosted an internationally acclaimed series of Historical Clinicopathological Conferences in Baltimore. These have generated over a score of peer-reviewed articles along with *Post Mortem: Solving History's Great Medical Mysteries,* the present book's prequel. In 2010, the American College of Physicians honored him with its Nicholas E. Davies Award for Scholarly Activities in the Humanities and History of Medicine, recognizing him as one of today's most accomplished medical historians.

Index